"All the yoga in the world will not stop us from getting older, but it can help us approach the journey with more grace, agility, and assuredness. Baxter Bell and Nina Zolotow show us how in *Yoga for Healthy Aging*. Their conversational style and gentle humor make their comprehensive medical knowledge and yoga teaching wisdom easily accessible to everyone—from beginning students to advanced teachers. And I love that they've given us concrete ways of *celebrating* who we are—instead of dreading what we fear we'll become—with each passing decade. A true gift for *all* ages."

—LINDA SPARROWE, author of *The Woman's Book of Yoga and Health* and *Yoga at Home*

"Thank you, Baxter and Nina, for creating this important yoga gem, which both allows us to refine our practice to be a boon to our health as we age and to create a sharper lens through which to know ourselves."

—RODNEY YEE, author of *Moving Toward Balance*

"Baxter Bell and Nina Zolotow share a wealth of information on using yoga safely to age with greater flexibility, strength, balance, and grace, both physically and psychologically. This user-friendly book will be a gift to yoga practitioners (and would-be practitioners), as well as those who teach them."

—TIMOTHY MCCALL, MD, author of *Yoga as Medicine*

"We might imagine from the title that this is a book only for the seniors among us. But in fact, the practices and supporting material will benefit both young and old alike. It will help the former establish a solid foundation for their future well-being and teach the latter how to maintain that well-being long into their 'golden' years."

—RICHARD ROSEN, author of *Yoga FAQ*

YOGA FOR HEALTHY AGING

A Guide to Lifelong Well-Being

Baxter Bell, MD
Nina Zolotow

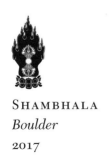

SHAMBHALA
Boulder
2017

Shambhala Publications, Inc.
4720 Walnut Street
Boulder, Colorado 80301
www.shambhala.com

9 8 7 6 5 4 3 2 1

FIRST EDITION
Printed in the United States of America

♾ This edition is printed on acid-free paper that meets the
American National Standards Institute z39.48 Standard.
♻ Shambhala makes every effort to print on recycled paper.
For more information please visit www.shambhala.com.

Distributed in the United States by Penguin Random House LLC
and in Canada by Random House of Canada Ltd

Designed by Steve Dyer

LIBRARY OF CONGRESS CATALOGING-IN-PUBLICATION DATA

Names: Bell, Baxter, author. | Zolotow, Nina, author.
Title: Yoga for healthy aging: a guide to lifelong well-being /
Baxter Bell, MD, Nina Zolotow.
Description: Boulder: Shambhala, 2017. | Includes index.
Identifiers: LCCN 2017004712 | ISBN 9781611803853 (paperback)
subjects: LCSH: Hatha yoga—Popular works. | Aging—Physiological
Aspects—Popular works. | BISAC: HEALTH & FITNESS / Yoga. |
SELF-HELP / Aging.
Classification: LCC RA781.7 .B43 2017 | DDC 613.7/046—dc23
LC record available at https://lccn.loc.gov/2017004712

CONTENTS

ACKNOWLEDGMENTS

When we got together to go over the list of people who had helped us with this book, we were amazed, humbled, and ever so grateful. There were so many of them! We are very fortunate indeed to know so many people who have a solid expertise in science, medicine, or health care combined with a deep appreciation of yoga.

We need to start first by thanking Dave O'Neal, senior editor at Shambhala Publications, for "discovering" us. It really was like the movies. At the end of our first Yoga for Healthy Aging intensive, one of the attendees—who we only knew at that point as "Dave"—approached Nina with his business card saying that if she really did want someone to pay her to write a book (something she had joked about during class), he'd be interested. Thank you so much, Dave, for appreciating our work and believing in us!

Special thanks are also due to Bradford Gibson, PhD, and Rammohan Rao, PhD, both from the Buck Institute for Research on Aging. Brad was there for us from the beginning, helping us to create our blog and teaching us about what is known—and what is not known—about aging. And when it came time to write the book, Brad helped Nina write the first chapter and reviewed the entire book for scientific accuracy and clarity. Ram, a neuroscientist, joined our team on the blog in year two as our expert on brain health as well as on several aspects of yoga. Our chapter on brain health wouldn't have been possible without him, as it is partly based on information we learned from him. He also reviewed the chapter after it was written for scientific accuracy.

Besides Brad and Ram, we had a whole team of experts who helped us out with their careful reviews of chapters that focused on their areas of expertise. So thanks to: Dilip Sarkar, MD, for reviewing the chapter on heart and cardiovascular system health; Laurie Baccash, physical therapist, for reviewing the chapters on strength, flexibility, balance, and agility; Matthew J. Taylor, physical therapist, for reviewing the chapters on strength and flexibility; Wayne Diamond, physical therapist, for reviewing the chapters on balance and agility; and Daniel Libby, PhD, for reviewing the chapter on stress management.

Thanks also to Anita Carstensen, MD, who took the time to review our long chapter on yoga for medical conditions, which, in the end, we could not include because, well, we were a bit overambitious about the initial scope of this book.

We also need to thank all our friends and members of the Yoga for Healthy Aging community who contributed their personal stories to our book, helping us to vividly illustrate how powerful yoga is for real life. We appreciate your openness and honesty—the fact that you were willing to tell the unvarnished truth is what made your stories so compelling—and the time you took to write for us. Here they are in alphabetical order by first name, with the name they wanted us to use: CJ Keller, Veterans Yoga Project Ambassador; Anita; Dan Libby, Veterans Yoga Project (for forwarding two veteran stories); Debbie Cabusas; Ellen Pechman; Elizabeth D.; Elizabeth Ann Gibbs; Evelyn Zak; Jill Satterfield; Mary Ann Avallone-O'Gorman; Melitta; Nina Rook; and Victor Dubin.

Thanks also to Bonnie, Carol, Jim, Judie, Krista, and Ramona for their stories about how yoga helped them with various medical conditions—we loved all those stories, though we couldn't use them in the end. We're saving them up, though!

Although our colleagues Dr. Timothy McCall and Shari Ser did not contribute directly to the book, we have learned so much from them over the years that we want to thank them for all they taught us—the book wouldn't be the same without you. And words cannot express our gratitude to our longtime teacher, Donald Moyer. Donald, so much of this book reflects knowledge that we gained from you, both about the asana practice and about what being a "yogi" really means.

Whew! All that was just about the words in the book, but a yoga book is pretty useless without photographs. Our photographer, Melina Meza, who is also a longtime yoga teacher and a certified Yoga for Healthy Aging teacher, really put her heart and soul into our project! Thank you so much, Melina, for taking such care to get each photo of every pose exactly right—some angles were quite tricky. And thank you to our model, Sandy Carmellini, who, like Melina, is a longtime yoga teacher and certified Yoga for Healthy Aging teacher. Thank you, Sandy, for the beautiful work you did in performing the poses, for your enthusiasm for our four different versions of every pose, and your patience throughout a demanding photo shoot.

Finally, thanks to Beth Frankl, our editor; Breanna Locke, Beth's assistant editor; and everyone else at Shambhala Publications for turning our text and photos into this beautiful book.

PART ONE

HOW TO PRACTICE YOGA FOR HEALTHY AGING

What Is Yoga for Healthy Aging?

FOR US, THE LIFE STORY OF OUR FRIEND MELITTA'S MOTHER, Nancy, personifies "healthy aging." Born in San Francisco on December 12, 1921, she died on August 27, 2015, at the age of 93. Nancy was very active all of her life. She played sports in school and was the shot put and discus champion at her high school and college. She loved skiing, sailing, hiking, horseback riding—all things outdoors—and worked as a wrangler at ranches around California. Even in her last years, she power walked every morning along the beach with her buddies Elaine and Ellen. When she started having back problems with spinal stenosis, Melitta gave her a yoga mat and some back-care yoga poses to do. Nancy did them faithfully every morning and was so pleased when they really improved her back.

Nancy also loved traveling and during her lifetime, she went around the world, visiting every continent. In 2011, she returned to Turkey, her favorite country, and in 2012, she took her last safari in Africa. She then gave up long-haul touring, although she continued to travel within the US to spend time with family.

Nancy volunteered at her church until about age 91, and she had a rich network of friends and family. She lived independently in her apartment until her last few days. At age 90, she made her own decision to stop driving. Although she didn't have any hired help, her friend Elaine took her shopping after she stopped driving.

It was only in the last year of her life that Nancy began to slow down, and at that time she and Melitta discussed her fear of decline—and Melitta's fear of her decline. In July 2015, she had surgery for a bile duct blockage. Then, in August 2015, she had emergency surgery for gallstones, but she also developed sepsis. Although the doctors "threw all the antibiotics" they could at her, her organs were failing, so the family followed her directives and discontinued care. When Melitta got to the hospital, Nancy was still conscious but unable to speak because she was intubated. In the joking way they had with each other, Melitta said, "It must be bad if I am here." Nancy laughed as best she could. She died two days later, with her children holding her as she passed on.

We'll come back to this story later when we discuss in detail what healthy aging means to us, and why yoga is such a powerful tool for fostering it. But for now, let's take a look at what aging itself actually is.

What Is Aging?

All living things age, and every species has a natural, built-in life span. Although giant tortoises and koi carp can live up to 200 years, the average life span of a human being is around 79 years. A cat lives to around 20, a dog to around 10, a mouse to around 2, a worm to only 10–30 days, and the infamous mayfly only lives a single day. But, no matter how brief their life span is, all of these living things go through a natural aging process (yes, even worms get all wrinkly in their old age), similar to the ones that we ourselves go through.

The formal definition of aging is "the process of a system's deterioration over time." From our perspective as human beings, this means that as we move through time and get older, our bodies just don't work as well as they did when we were younger. We'll be discussing this in some detail in chapters 3 through 8.

Now you may think that with all the scientific breakthroughs of the last century, from determining the structure of atoms and the properties of subatomic particles to mapping the human genome, we would have a pretty good understanding of why all living things age and how it happens.

Nina's husband, Brad, who is a medical researcher with a PhD in biochemistry, had this same impression when he started working sixteen years ago at the Buck Institute for Research on Aging. On his first day, as he entered the elegant I. M. Pei building on the top of a beautiful hill in the Marin County countryside, he was excited to start applying his knowledge of chemistry and technology to slowing down aging and eliminating age-related diseases. Instead, he was amazed to find out that there were many different—and often conflicting—theories on aging. Here's how he described it:

> As I examined theories such as the free radical theory of aging to antagonistic pleiotropy, it became readily apparent that this was still early days of this discipline. While many of the processes described in these competing theories seemed plausible, they couldn't all be correct! So working in this field was going to be much more confusing—and interesting—than I had originally imagined.

More recently, he and some of his colleagues have come to believe that instead of any one single cause of aging, there are actually multiple contributors, such as inflammation, stress, and molecular damage, which are all linked to each other in very complex ways. As a result, a new field called "geroscience" has emerged to identify how these different processes intertwine and interact to cause what we experience as "aging."

Just to give you a general idea, here's an illustration that shows what most geroscientists now consider to be the "seven pillars of aging."

If this looks complicated and overwhelming, it is! But the bottom line is that it's going to take a lot more work and discoveries to reach a full understanding of what aging is and how we might intervene in the aging process.

However, even though scientists have not yet discovered how to slow, stop, or reverse aging, scientific studies done on people who lived long and healthy lives provide us with solid evidence that there are many steps you can take to improve your health and the quality of your life as you age. For example, we know regular exercise, stress management, and a healthy diet can have a huge effect on your physical, mental, and emotional well-being.

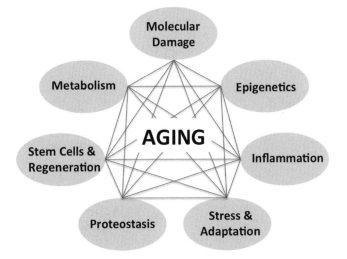

In addition there are many serious diseases for which aging is a major risk factor, including heart disease, stroke, and osteoporosis. The good news is that for these and many other diseases there are actions you can take to help prevent them from developing or to slow down their progression.

Although people still dream about slowing aging to extend human longevity (and scientists are exploring some possibilities to do so), we have no idea how long this will take or even if it's possible in our lifetimes. What you can do here and now is to foster well-being throughout the life span you do have. And that's what we mean by "healthy aging."

ABOUT HEALTHY AGING

As more people are living longer and fewer are dying young from diseases caused by infections or insufficient food, exponentially more middle-aged and elderly people are suffering from chronic noninfectious diseases that used to be rare or unknown.

— Daniel Lieberman, *The Story of the Human Body*

In his book *The Story of the Human Body: Evolution, Health, and Disease,* Daniel Lieberman describes how human beings evolved to live a hunter-gatherer lifestyle, one that includes being very physically active (we evolved for endurance walking and running), eating lots of fruits and vegetables and other unprocessed foods (rather than quickly metabolized high-processed foods), and experiencing stress only in short, acute bursts rather than chronically. He says that because our bodies did not evolve to handle being sedentary for years on end, regular consumption of a surplus of calories, and/or a chronically stressful lifestyle, the result is an increase in serious diseases and chronic illnesses, such as heart disease, stroke, cancer, type 2 diabetes, and osteoporosis.

That's why for the past several years we've been on a mission to teach people how yoga can help prevent much of the ill health, disability, and suffering that has become associated with aging in developed countries. To illustrate what we mean, let's revisit the life story we told in the beginning of this chapter about Nancy, who lived to 93. Her story exemplifies what we see as the three essential concepts of healthy aging: compressed morbidity, independence, and equanimity.

Compressed Morbidity

This is the time out of our life spans that we spend in ill health. Obviously, we'd like to keep this as short as possible. Nancy had a lifetime of excellent health, with some slowing down and her only serious problems limited to her last year of life. No doubt, a lifetime of regular exercise and engaging in activities that gave her life meaning helped make that possible.

We guess it's rather obvious, but your life span is the period of time during which you are alive. However, that life span could include any number of years spent in poor health. Right now, although life spans in first-world countries have increased significantly due to better nutrition and modern medicine, middle-aged and elderly people in first-world countries can suffer many years of ill health before they die. This period of ill health is referred to as "morbidity." Now let's do a little bit of simple math:

Life span − morbidity = health span

To put it into words, your "health span" is equal to your life span minus the amount of time you spend in ill health. This is the period in your life during which you are generally healthy and free from serious or chronic illness. When we talk about healthy aging, we don't mean increasing your life span or your longevity. Instead, we mean doing what you can to keep your health span as long as possible (and the period of time you spend in ill health near the end of your life as short as possible). To make this happen, you'll need to combine regular exercise with stress management practices because both are necessary for maintaining overall physical health and brain health and preventing serious stress-related diseases, such as heart disease and stroke.

Independence

Independence means being able to live on your own and engage in the activities that you love and that give your life meaning. Nancy was not only able to stay in her home until the end of her life, she was able to maintain her very active life almost until the end, including traveling around the world, walking on the beach, volunteering at church, and spending time with friends and family.

When medical professionals talk about maintaining independence, they typically focus on our ability to live in our own homes and take care of ourselves as long as possible. So they tend to focus on basic daily self-care activities, such as dressing, going to the toilet, getting up and down from a chair, doing light housework, and so on. But we think they've been overlooking other important aspects of staying independent.

The first is the ability to continue to do what we love. This can include physical activities, such as cycling, hiking, doing construction projects, or gardening, but also includes activities that get us out of the house and into the world, such as attending concerts and plays, art exhibits, and poetry readings, or joining family and other social gatherings.

For many, being independent also means being able to do the work that gives shape to their days and keeps their intellects fully engaged, whether that means writing poetry or playing music, keeping up with a law or science career, or teaching in their area of expertise. For others, the ability to dedicate themselves to a cause, whether large or small, is what makes life worth living. This can include being politically active, volunteering at a school, food bank, or animal shelter, helping people learn to read and write, or even acting as a caregiver for family members or others.

So for a truly independent life, you'll need to maintain a combination of four physical skills—strength, flexibility, balance, and agility—which will allow you to be mobile and capable out in the world at large. You'll also need to maintain brain health and emotional stability so you can take care of yourself and continue to participate in the activities that give your life meaning.

Equanimity

Equanimity means being able to face difficulty and handle challenges with balance and grace. Although we don't know much about how she faced earlier challenges, we think it's worth considering how Nancy dealt with the challenges of getting older. It sounds like she faced them head-on! She realistically decided to stop overseas travel and driving when the time was right. And she was able to discuss her fears of decline and to confront her death. That allowed her to leave directives for her family and to die on her own terms. Finally, being able to laugh at her daughter's joke at the very end sounds like she was able to stay engaged in life and family for all of her days. How beautiful!

Although our mission is to explore all the ways that yoga can help you extend your health span and stay independent as you age, we recognize that there may be times when serious challenges arise. For even if we can extend our health spans, unless we die very suddenly, we will have to go through poor health at some point. And even if we can prolong our independence into old age, eventually we are likely to need help from others, however briefly. In addition, even if we are ourselves blessed with long and healthy lives, we'll all have to deal with losing people we love and many other types of difficulties. So being able to handle the challenges that life throws at us with balance and grace is crucial. That's why we believe that cultivating equanimity is the most important aspect of healthy aging. To cultivate equanimity, you'll need to manage chronic stress, maintain emotional stability, and learn new ways of thinking about your life and your place in the world.

Nina Rook, whose life was thrown off track when her marriage ended and her older sister, with whom she had decided to spend her later years, died suddenly, says:

> I feel that yoga helps me take some responsibility for my own well-being, while acknowledging my lack of control. It also reinforces my ability to exult in the present, to draw energy from whatever I am experiencing. The toolbox that is so valuable in maintaining health also helps me to maintain the mental agility to cope with whatever the fates sling at me, for as long as possible.[1]

Well said, Nina Rook! We agree. And that's exactly why we're such advocates for yoga—we believe it can help with all three aspects of healthy aging. Next we'll look at what yoga is and how it can help you work toward achieving these goals.

WHAT IS YOGA?

Before we explain why yoga is such a powerful solution for fostering healthy aging, we need to define what we mean by "yoga." After all, yoga means different things to different people. Many Americans—including doctors who recommend yoga to their patients—think yoga is "just stretching." In fact, when Nina started taking yoga classes, she didn't have a clue what yoga was. When one of her coworkers at a software company said that his wife could teach an on-site "exercise class," she decided to give it a go. On that first day of class, when they were all standing around in their exercise clothes, the teacher asked them to start by taking "Mountain Pose," with their big toes together and their heels slightly apart. Just standing that way felt so wonderful that Nina thought, "Whatever this is, this is for me!" Her experience of falling in love with the asana practice (the practice of physical postures) without knowing anything about the rest of yoga is actually very common.

In fact, yoga as an exercise system is only a very small part of a much larger tradition and a very recent development in the long history of yoga. Although yoga is arguably thousands of years old, what yogis were doing back in the early days had nothing at all to do with Tree Pose or Sun Salutations. Early yogis were spiritual seekers, with the aim of understanding the ultimate truths of reality. In order to pursue this goal, they developed practices, including meditation and *pranayama* (breath control), to allow them to concentrate and free their minds from distraction.

Although the original yogis were Hindus with religious goals of achieving "union with the divine," the yoga techniques they developed for quieting the mind were so effective and their teachings about the nature of the mind and the causes of human suffering were so profound that yoga was adopted by other religions, including Buddhism, Jainism, and Sikhism. (And, of course, today people of many other religions—or no religion at all—also practice yoga.) The classic yoga text from 500 to 400 B.C.E., the Bhagavad Gita, defines yoga as follows:

Yoga is evenness of mind—a peace that is ever the same.[2]

Naturally as yoga spread throughout the East and among very different peoples, it evolved in a myriad of ways. Yoga was eventually codified by Patanjali between 150 and 200 C.E. in The Yoga Sutras, a text that we still use as a reference today. However, the school of yoga summarized in this work was just one of the many that existed during that era.

> Yoga is an art, a science, and a philosophy. It touches the life of man at every level, physical, mental, and spiritual.
>
> —B. K. S. Iyengar, *Light on the Yoga Sūtras of Patañjali*

It wasn't until tantra and hatha yoga developed (approximately 800 or 900 C.E.) that various physical practices, including yoga postures, became essential aspects of yoga. Even then, although the Hatha Yoga Pradipika (1200–1300 C.E.) mentions the existence of eighty-four poses, or asanas, it mentions only fifteen by name. The aim of practicing these postures was to train the yogi to be able to remain comfortably seated in meditation for long periods of time.

It was really only in the twentieth century that pivotal figures such as T. K. V. Krishnamacharya and B. K. S. Iyengar developed the modern yoga poses as we now know them. These teachers consciously expanded the repertoire of traditional poses, blending techniques from British and Chinese gymnastics, European fitness programs, and Indian wrestling with classic hatha yoga postures. They also developed the use of yoga props, with the aim of making yoga accessible to ordinary people, and they adapted the yoga poses for treating medical conditions. (If you're disappointed that the modern asana practice was essentially invented in the early twentieth century, take a moment to acknowledge the genius of those teachers— the system they developed was so effective and powerful that it spread throughout the world.) During this period, for many practitioners in the West, yoga became completely disassociated from its spiritual aspects and the asana practice was adopted solely as an exercise system.

Trying to cover thousands of years of yoga history in a few paragraphs means oversimplifying quite a bit. But one way to think about it is this: yoga is a collection of techniques and concepts adopted from both ancient and contemporary India that allows you to take care of your body as well as your soul.

The first time Baxter tried yoga was when he was still working as a medical doctor in a busy family practice. He had a classic "monkey mind" back then and was constantly reviewing and worrying about his work decisions, dealing with the immediate intense crises of the present day, or planning his next short- and long-term adventures. While his stiff, inflexible body was really challenged by the yoga practice, it was the effect of the final Relaxation Pose that surprised him. His busy, worrying, planning mind actually took a break, if just for a few moments. When it was over and he sat up, he felt a profound and welcomed sense of peace and calm that was rare for him. He had just discovered a discipline that could satisfy his need for physicality and also rest and refresh his mind and spirit!

Your Yoga Toolbox

Because the history of yoga is so long and rich, we have a very large collection of techniques and concepts—let's call them tools—to draw on for this book. We've chosen to focus on just a select few: the ones that we believe are most valuable for fostering healthy aging and lifelong well-being. It's like those beautiful starter toolboxes we sometimes drool over at the hardware store—even though there is nothing esoteric or fancy in there, the box contains a complete set of solid tools that you could use to build just about anything.

YOGA POSES (ASANAS). From among the hundreds of modern yoga poses, we selected a subset of essential poses for you to practice. These versatile and accessible poses will help you maintain your physical health. You can use them to cultivate strength, flexibility, balance, and agility—our four essential physical skills for staying healthy and independent as you age. You can also use them to cultivate cardiovascular health and brain health, and to reduce chronic stress. All of these benefits help to foster a longer health span.

Our essential yoga poses will also help you cultivate equanimity and stay emotionally balanced. You can use these poses to quiet your nervous system when you're stressed or angry, uplift yourself when you're blue, or just experience deep relaxation whenever you need it.

These essential poses are easy to do, and you'll be using them throughout the book as you learn to practice yoga for healthy aging. For those of you who are stiff, weak, or have physical problems, we provide variations and options for using props that make the poses accessible to everyone.

MEDITATION. Your toolbox includes a variety of meditation techniques so you can experiment and find the ones that work best for you. If you've never meditated before, we'll teach you how—it's easier than you think. In addition to traditional seated meditation, you'll learn to use mindfulness techniques in your yoga sessions to practice moving meditation. The original yogis used meditation techniques to quiet the mind, develop concentration, and learn about habitual thought patterns, all of which help cultivate equanimity. You can also use meditation to reduce stress, build brain strength, and set an intention. All of these benefits will help you maintain the health of your body and mind at the same time that you cultivate spiritual well-being.

BREATH PRACTICES (PRANAYAMA). These simple tools are surprisingly powerful. You can use basic breath awareness to reduce stress levels or as a focus for meditation. Our structured breath practices provide you with the ability to calm yourself when you're stressed, anxious, or angry; energize yourself when you're lethargic; uplift yourself when you're feeling blue; or balance yourself when you need only subtle calming or stimulating.

These tools will help you manage stress, maintain emotional stability, and cultivate equanimity.

PHILOSOPHY. We'll introduce you to two of the most influential yoga texts—the Bhagavad Gita and The Yoga Sutras—and we'll delve into some of the essential yoga concepts that we believe have the power to change your approach to aging, well-being, and life. Every day in Western cultures we're bombarded with advertising that tells us that in order to be happy, we must buy more and achieve more. The wisdom of yoga will provide you with a different way of thinking. Although the world has changed in many ways since the classic yoga texts were written, human nature stays the same. So the original goal of yoga—peace of mind—is one that many of us still aspire to. Studying yoga philosophy and learning to practice its tenets will allow you to prevent chronic stress from developing in the first place and can help you cultivate new ways of interacting with the people in your life and the world at large.

> Just as this is not the best of all possible worlds, your body is not the best of all possible bodies. But it's the only one you'll ever have, and it's worth enjoying, nurturing, and protecting.
>
> —Daniel Lieberman, *The Story of the Human Body*

HOW TO PRACTICE YOGA FOR HEALTHY AGING

Although we advise you to practice yoga regularly with the goals of attaining a longer health span and maintaining your independence, we also believe it is important to keep in mind that results are never guaranteed. As we said earlier, the basic processes underlying human aging are inescapable, at least as we currently understand them. So we feel that at the same time that you work toward staying healthy by using the tools in your yoga toolbox, you should try to let go of all thoughts of success or failure and simply focus on your practice.

This is the basic yogic attitude that is conveyed in the Bhagavad Gita:

> Self-possessed, resolute, act
> without any thoughts of results,
> open to success or failure.
> This equanimity is yoga.[3]

Taking this approach means that even while you are actively engaged in working toward your goals of lengthening your health span and maintaining your independence—or any other goals you set for yourself—you also practice acceptance of your life in the real world as it unfolds. Cultivating equanimity through a combination of active engagement and acceptance is what provides you with lifelong well-being, as you navigate through all the stages of your life.

Because this is such an essential concept for practicing yoga for healthy aging—and for anyone, of any age, who wants to experience peace of mind—we discuss it in depth in chapters 10 and 11. But for now, the best place to begin is to start practicing. As B. K. S. Iyengar says:

> Words cannot convey the total value of yoga. It has to be experienced.[4]

Preparing to Practice

BEFORE WE RECOMMEND YOGA POSES AND SEQUENCES FOR YOU to practice, we want to make sure you know how to customize your yoga practice for your particular needs. One of the most important benefits of practicing yoga at home is that no matter what you're going through you can do the practice that's right for you on any given day.

This chapter provides common sense guidelines that we recommend you follow as you start to practice yoga for healthy aging. As longtime home practitioners, we follow these guidelines ourselves when we practice at home and when we attend public classes, and we encourage our students to do the same. The chapter covers the following:

How to practice our sequences. Our book is full of simple, accessible yoga sequences you can practice on your own at home. Before you get started, we'll provide you with some tips for how you can get the most out of these practices.

Using yoga props. For those of you who are not already using yoga props, we'll discuss why yoga props are beneficial, which ones you'll need to do our practices, and how to use common household objects for props.

How to rest. As important as it is to challenge yourself, it's also vital to know when to rest—and how to rest.

Customizing your home practice. Because everyone has different desires and concerns, we'll describe how you can adapt our sequences to your particular needs.

Safety guidelines. Although yoga is generally safe, there are several steps you can take to ensure you're not taking unnecessary risks.

Contraindications. For those of you with medical conditions—whether they're temporary or ongoing—we'll let you know which types of movements you should be avoiding.

ABOUT OUR SEQUENCES

This book contains many sequences of poses for you to practice on your own. For those of you who are not experienced practitioners or who are not familiar with some of our variations of the poses, we have described every pose in our sequences—our essential yoga poses—in detail in part 2.

For all essential yoga poses, we have four variations. The first variation is always the classic version (done without props) of the pose. Then we provide three more accessible variations. Sometimes the accessible variations use props, which help make the pose safer, more comfortable, or just plain doable. Other times we simply change up the pose. An example of this is Side Plank Pose. The first two variations of the classic pose don't use props but a slightly different shape instead (the first with a different foot position and the second with a different arm position). The final variation reorients the pose completely, so you're standing upright instead of balancing on the edge of your feet.

If a sequence in our book specifies a particular version number of a pose, then you should do that version if it's accessible to you. However, if we just give the pose name without a version number, then feel free to do whichever version you prefer.

In addition to our essential yoga poses, which are static poses (you hold the pose for an extended period of time), our sequences also include dynamic poses, in which you move in and out of the pose with your breath, and flow sequences, in which you move through several linked poses with your breath. See "Dynamic Poses and Flow Sequences" in part 2 for photos of the individual movements in our dynamic poses and flow sequences, along with breathing instructions.

Timing

All of our sequences include recommended timings for holding the poses. For active poses that you hold for two minutes or less, we recommend that you count your breaths instead of using a timer. So you'll first need to do some experimenting with a watch or timer to find how many breaths you take in gentle and active poses.

IN GENTLE POSES. Start by counting how many breaths per minute you typically take in a gentler pose, such as Easy Sitting Twist or Reclined Leg Stretch. Then, for all gentle poses in our sequences, you can simply count the appropriate amount of breaths. For example, if you take twelve breaths per minute in a gentle pose, you'd hold the pose for twenty-four breaths to time yourself for two minutes in a pose.

IN ACTIVE POSES. Next count how many breaths per minute you typically take in a more physically demanding pose, such as Extended Side Angle Pose, Plank Pose, or Warrior 3 Pose. Then for all the more demanding poses in our sequences, you can simply count the appropriate number of breaths. For example, if you take sixteen breaths per minute in a demanding pose, you would hold the pose for eight breaths to time yourself for thirty seconds in a pose.

For holds that are longer than two minutes, such as for restorative yoga poses or Relaxation Pose, we recommend you use a timer, such as the one on your watch or phone. That way, you will be free to concentrate on the particular focus for that pose (and this will also help prevent you from falling asleep and staying too long in the pose).

Finally, if the recommended timing for a pose seems too long or too short for you, please feel free to change the timing to one that's better for you. And if the sequence itself is too long, you can do fewer repetitions of poses that repeat, skip poses entirely, or stop at a place that feels right for you (although ending with the final resting pose). See "Customizing Your Practice" on page 21 for more ways to customize our sequences.

How Often to Practice a Sequence

If there's a particular sequence in our book that you love or that focuses on an area that you'd like to work on (such as strength, balance, stress management, or cardiovascular health), you can practice it up to three times a week. For other practice days, we recommend that you mix it up by practicing sequences from other parts of our book. Here's why:

- Doing the same poses in the same order every single day means that you run the risk of repetitive stress injuries. That's not yoga's fault; it's just the nature of the human body. Any joint is vulnerable if you overuse it. For example, too many forward bends can cause back strain, just as too much gardening can.

- You'll be missing out on yoga's other benefits. It's like eating the same thing every day—even if you're eating healthy food, you'll still be missing out on some of your important nutrients. For example, if the only sequence you do is an active one, you'll be missing out on the many benefits provided by restorative or quieting sequences. Or, if the only balance pose you do throughout the week is Tree Pose, you'll miss out on challenging your balance in other important ways.

- Mixing it up keeps you from getting into a rut, which can lead to getting bored with your practice. Moving out of your comfort zone in your practice is the best way to keep your mind stimulated (good for brain health!) and to learn something about your habits and thought patterns while you're at it.

USING YOGA PROPS

If you have never used yoga props before, you may be wondering why we're so committed to them. You may be thinking that they just make practicing more complicated, or you may even feel like using them is cheating. (Yes, we've heard those things before.) So for those of you who need a little convincing, these are our reasons for using props:

Props keep you safe. Using a prop can help prevent injuries caused by overstretching or misalignment. For people who have trouble reaching the floor—whether due to anatomy (short arms) or lack of flexibility—using a prop in, for example, Triangle Pose or Standing Forward Bend, can make the difference between overstretching your hamstrings and keeping them healthy. For people who are stiff or have back problems, using a prop can reduce physical stress. For example, version 4 of Reclined Twist adds a bolster to decrease stress on your lower back and make the pose more comfortable for those who have tight hips.

Props stabilize you. For people who have balance problems or who lack leg, knee, or hip strength, using props in standing poses can keep you from falling. You can use a wall (with a foot or hand on the wall) or a chair (with a hand on the chair seat or back). Even using a block to support your hand can help stabilize you in the pose.

Props make breathing easier. Using a prop to achieve a healthy alignment—one in which your spine maintains its natural curves and your chest is open—helps you to take deep and easy breaths. For example, if your hips are tight, sitting on a block or folded blanket allows you to maintain an upright posture, rather than hunching your back and collapsing your chest. Using props can also help reduce pain in a pose (e.g., foot or knee pain in Hero Pose), allowing you to be more comfortable, which makes breathing easier, too.

Props let you heal. After you injure yourself or experience illness or surgery, using props allows you to gradually restore strength and flexibility to a challenged area. For example, someone recovering from a wrist injury could practice Downward-Facing Dog Pose with hands on the wall, then hands on a chair, and then hands on blocks while moving through the healing process.

Props let you relax. Without props, there wouldn't be restorative yoga! In restorative poses, the props allow you to take the shape of a pose, such as a backbend, twist, or forward bend, without muscular effort so you can stay in the pose for long periods of time and relax deeply. Using props in more active poses that otherwise push you to your absolute limits allows you to be comfortable—or at least be *more* comfortable—while still obtaining the benefits of the pose.

Props empower you. When you're ready to progress beyond the basics, props can enable you to take the first baby steps toward a challenging pose. For example, practicing Warrior 3 Pose or Side Plank Pose with a wall is a good way to start working toward the classic versions of the poses.

Props enable all of us. No matter what shape you're in—even if you can't get down to the floor, can't stand up, or can't move parts of your body—props allow you to take the shape of a pose and obtain the benefits of stretching, moving your joints, and breathing mindfully. With yoga props, there is always a way.

Recommended Props

Before practicing our sequences, we recommend that you put together the following basic set of yoga props. You don't necessarily have to run out and spend a lot of money on "official" yoga props. Often there is something in the house that will work just fine: a sturdy dining room chair, an old belt or tie to use as a strap, the cotton Mexican blanket you bought as a souvenir, and thick old textbooks, wrapped in duct tape for makeshift blocks!

One yoga mat (a thin sticky mat, not a padded exercise mat). Although a yoga mat is not strictly necessary for standing poses (especially if

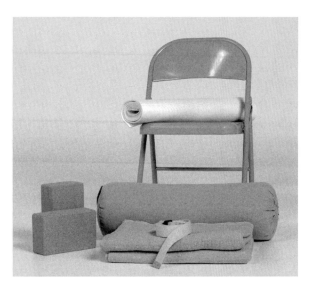

you're practicing on a wood floor), it can be very useful for providing some cushioning and for keeping other props from slipping around.

Two same-sized yoga blocks (wood, cork, or foam). If you decide to use books instead of blocks, just make sure they're the same size, so when you are using both at the same time, you aren't propping yourself unevenly.

One eight-foot yoga strap (preferably with a buckle). For our essential yoga poses, any kind of belt or tie will do, such as the belt on a bathrobe.

One round yoga bolster. If you have two densely woven blankets, you can "fake" a round bolster by rolling the first blanket into a firm roll and then rolling it up inside the second blanket.

Two densely woven single blankets. In a pinch, you can use multiple bath towels to substitute for a yoga blanket.

One sturdy chair, with an opening in the chair back. If you can't find a chair with an opening in the back and want to support your shins on the chair, you can turn the chair sideways.

RESTING BETWEEN POSES

Sometimes when you're in the middle of practicing a sequence that is challenging or have just done a particularly challenging pose, you might be ready for a short rest before continuing on with your next pose. Recognizing that you need to rest is actually an advanced skill because it means you have the experience, understanding, courage, and confidence to know when enough is enough for your body and mind. If you are suffering from fatigue, a recent cold or flu, or recovering from or dealing with treatment for serious illness, the brief rest can allow you to safely do a practice, while providing some true rest during your pauses.

Here are some suggestions of ways to rest, based on the type of pose you were previously doing:

- After a supine pose (on your back), rest in Relaxation Pose.
- After a prone pose (on your belly), rest in Child's Pose.
- After a seated pose, such as a twist or forward bend, rest in Easy Sitting Pose.
- After a standing pose, rest in Mountain Pose.
- After an inverted pose or backbend, come down into Child's Pose or Relaxation Pose.

In addition to providing you with the rest, your break can serve as an opportunity to do a "pose assessment" in which you evaluate the effects—positive, negative, or neutral—of your practice so far. One easy way to do this is to notice how the pose you just practiced affected your breathing. Did it calm it, speed it up, agitate it, or slow it down? From there, consider other physical sensations you feel as objectively as possible. Ask yourself, "Where do I feel sensation now? Am I feeling a stretch sensation, a strong muscle contraction, or unwanted pain? Is there a sense of effort still lingering? Am I experiencing fatigue or weakness, vitality or aliveness? What is the effect on my mood or emotions?"

Your pose assessment not only lets you notice the immediate effects of the last pose but may also guide you to your next pose. Even with our sequences, you can always choose to skip over a pose or add in another one. And when you create your own sequences, you will be able to ensure that they are aligned with the intention you set for your practice. As you notice openness, strength, or vulnerability, the feedback may send you in new and unimagined directions that you could easily have missed if you practiced in a more automatic way.

CUSTOMIZING YOUR PRACTICE

One of the important advantages of practicing at home is being able to do the right practice for you—one that suits your particular needs and desires—on any given day. But if designing your own sequences from scratch is too overwhelming to consider, a good first step is to tinker a bit with a practice from our book (or elsewhere). It's simpler than you might imagine!

This section provides basic recommendations for customizing any practice to make it:

- More gentle
- More vigorous
- Shorter or longer
- Adapted to your particular limitations

Making a Practice More Gentle

You can make any practice more gentle by:

- Doing fewer repetitions of dynamic poses (e.g., doing three rounds of dynamic Warrior 2 Pose instead of six)

- Using shorter holds in static poses (e.g., holding Warrior 3 Pose for three breaths instead of six)
- Extending your time in restorative poses
- Skipping the most vigorous pose or poses in the sequence or replacing it or them with gentle or restorative poses
- Doing a resting pose (e.g., Relaxation Pose) between active poses

Making a Practice More Vigorous

You can take any practice except a restorative sequence and make it more vigorous by:

- Doing more repetitions of dynamic poses (e.g., doing ten rounds of dynamic Warrior 2 Pose instead of six)
- Extending your holds in static poses (e.g., holding Warrior 3 Pose for ten or twelve breaths instead of six) or repeating poses a second or third time instead of doing them only once
- Repeating a series of static poses an extra time
- Adding in any poses you feel are more vigorous for you, placing them after the warm-up poses and before the cool-down poses

Making a Practice Shorter or Longer

We all feel the time crunch now and then and, conversely, sometimes find that we have extra time on a given day. You can easily adjust the length of your practice depending on how much time you have to devote to it on any given day.

You can shorten a practice by:

- Doing fewer repetitions of dynamic poses
- Using shorter holds for static poses
- Eliminating any poses from the sequence that are less appealing today but keeping in at least some of the initial warm-up poses and at least one cool-down pose

You can lengthen a practice by:

- Lengthening the time you spend in some of the poses, either increasing the repetitions of dynamic poses or extending your holds in static or restorative poses
- Repeating your favorite pose or poses a few times
- Adding in more poses of the same type (e.g., adding in more

backbends in a backbend sequence or more strength-building poses in a strength-building sequence)

- Adding in a short meditation or breath practice that is not in the sequence
- Doing Relaxation Pose or another resting pose between poses
- Taking an extra-long time in Relaxation Pose

Adapting a Practice to Your Limitations

INJURY. If you have an injury you can still practice by adapting the individual poses to your limitations. For example, with a shoulder injury, you can keep your arms down at your sides in many standing poses or practice Half Downward-Facing Dog Pose instead of classic Downward-Facing Dog. You can simply skip those poses you cannot adapt. For example, skip Plank Pose if you have a shoulder injury. When you're in the acute and recovery phases of an injury, floor sequences and chair variations are good alternatives.

ILLNESS. When you are ill or recovering from an illness, focus on gentle, restorative practices until you recover. When you're ready for a more active practice, use our recommendations above to make your first active practice days easier.

DISABILITY. If you're working with a longer-term disability, adapt your practice as we described for an injury. Because you'll be practicing this way for a long period of time, it may also be worth getting special guidance from a skilled teacher for creative ways you can adapt various poses to your condition.

Have fun practicing and don't be afraid to get creative!

SAFETY GUIDELINES

Whether you're practicing yoga at home from our book or taking a class, we recommend that you use the following guidelines to practice wisely. That may mean there's a pose, group of poses, or practice you cannot or should not be doing, sometimes temporarily and sometimes permanently. This can be hard. It's natural to feel left out when other people in your class or other people you know are doing a pose that you cannot or should not do. It's also challenging for us longtime practitioners to say goodbye to poses that we used to be able to do. But rest assured that you are not missing out on anything essential. Regardless of your limitations, there are still effective ways to foster strength, flexibility, balance, and agility and to manage your stress levels. That's why we have four versions of every pose we recommend, as well as alternate poses to provide the same effects. And, of course, the experience of practicing an asana mindfully, as a moving meditation, is available to everyone, no matter your limitations (see chapter 10).

This is an opportunity for you to experiment with cultivating contentment (*santosha*) in a safe space. When you start to practice, gently remind yourself that you can be content with what you have and what you don't have. You'll then find that you can enjoy your time on the mat no matter which poses you can't do. Cultivating contentment in the yoga room will strengthen your equanimity muscles as you strengthen your physical ones. You can then take your experience of becoming content with what you have and what you don't have out into the world at large. (See chapter 11 for more information on contentment.)

Talk to Your Doctor

If you have had surgery or have a medical condition or an injury, explicitly ask your doctor or physical therapist which physical actions are safe for you and which are not. Don't wait for the medical professional to tell you! Some doctors often don't even consider that you may be going upside down or twisting yourself into a pretzel. Here are fifteen questions that we recommend you ask:

1. Can I go upside down?
2. Can I round my spine forward, backward, or side to side?
3. Can I twist my spine?
4. Can I cross my legs?
5. Can I put pressure on this or that part of my body, such as my knees or wrists?
6. Can I stand on one leg?
7. Can I practice in bare feet?
8. Is my recovery from this serious illness at a point where I can safely increase my physical activity?
9. Is it safe for me to do a vigorous practice where I am sweating and exerting myself?
10. Is it okay for me to hold standing poses, which require endurance and strength, for long periods of time?
11. Is it all right to stretch my injured tendon, ligament, or muscle now?
12. Would any of the medicine I am taking interfere with my practicing by making me dizzy, unfocused, distracted, off balance, or sleepy?

13. How long should I wait before returning to class or home practice?

14. After my surgery, how long do I wait before it is safe to stretch the area where my incision or scar is?

15. After my joint replacement or repair, is there a limit to my range of motion in certain directions that I should honor?

Acknowledge Your Limitations

Before starting to practice, take a moment to list any illnesses, conditions, or medical problems that might affect your ability to do certain poses or put you at risk. Some examples are osteoporosis/osteopenia, uncontrolled high blood pressure, diabetes, and lower back, knee, or hip pain. Then see "Appendix: Contraindications for Medical Conditions" to find out what types of poses you should not be doing with your particular condition. If you are unsure, ask your yoga teacher or health care professional.

If you have no medical problems but know that you are particularly stiff or weak or have problems with balance, you will be able to do some version of all the poses in this book. However, we recommend that you try the version of a pose that is easiest and has the most support first rather than starting with the classic version.

Use Props

Using props is never "cheating." In fact, using props when you need them is an essential part of practicing wisely. So if you know that a prop is important for your safety or comfort (to keep you from overstretching or falling or to use as padding for sensitive areas), go ahead and use it even if we have not specifically instructed you to do so.

Stay Balanced

If you are weak or have trouble with balance, use a prop, such as a chair or the wall, to stabilize yourself so that you don't fall over and can practice with confidence. For standing poses, you can practice with your back near a wall, with one foot against the wall, or with one hand on the wall. For example, for Warrior 2 Pose, try practicing either with your back near the wall or with your back heel on the wall.

Pay Attention to Pain

Learn to tell the difference between sensations that are potentially good for you, such as the healthy stretching of a muscle, and those that are potentially injurious, such as overstretching a tendon or ligament or compressing structures to the point of injury. (See "Healthy and Unhealthy Stretching Sensations" on page 58 for more information about healthy and unhealthy stretching sensations.) If you catch yourself moving into a sensation that feels dangerous or that you are concerned about, try backing off a bit, perhaps by reducing a stretch or by using a prop. If you can't back off for some reason or that doesn't help, come out of the pose and rest.

Listen to Your Breath

Although your breath may come more quickly in demanding poses, such as backbends or standing poses, gasping for breath indicates that you're overstressing yourself, so see if you can back out of the pose a bit, possibly by using a prop. If you can't back out for some reason or if doing that doesn't help you catch your breath, come out of the pose and rest.

Notice if you are holding your breath because this is a possible sign that you are becoming fearful or anxious or reacting to pain. If you find you are holding your breath, consciously relax your breathing.

Rest If You Need To

If you feel you've reached your limit in a pose, stop and take a rest. If you are suddenly sweating much more than normal, this could be a sign that you're overstressing yourself, and you should take the same precautions. You can then continue on when you are ready.

If you feel like you just can't finish the rest of a sequence, lie down in a comfortable Relaxation Pose (see "Relaxation Pose" on page 256). Don't just stop in the middle of a practice without cooling down.

Contraindications for Medical Conditions

Regardless of our age, the vast majority of us experience health problems at one time or another. Sometimes we've suffered a minor or major injury. Sometimes we're experiencing an illness, either temporary or chronic. Sometimes we're dealing with wear and tear on the body, such as arthritis. Although you can always practice some form of yoga no matter what your health status is, for certain medical conditions there are certain types of movements that you should not be making, as they could either aggravate your condition or perhaps even be risky for you.

In the appendix, we list the medical conditions for each type of movement that we recommend you avoid. If you don't know what the movement type means, see the follow-up tables and the section on inverted poses.

Generally, these contraindications are relative, which means that limited movements in that direction may still be possible for you. So start by trying a limited movement at first and allow feedback from your body to tell you whether you can take it further or whether you should stop doing the pose. Especially for painful areas, we recommend trying a non-weight-bearing movement first; if that is fine, try the same movement in a weight-bearing pose.

Yoga for Strength

SIX MONTHS BEFORE HER SIXTY-FIFTH BIRTHDAY, ELLEN PECHMAN started experiencing intense lower back pain. She especially had difficulty moving from sitting to standing, climbing and descending the staircases in her house, and walking in her neighborhood. A visit to the doctor led to a diagnosis of "irreversible stenosis" coupled with osteoporosis in two hip points. This is when she turned to her yoga teachers. She had been taking a yoga class once a week for several years, but after her diagnosis she began to practice yoga seriously. Because she had mild scoliosis, she started by studying with a teacher who specialized in yoga for scoliosis, learning how to use yoga poses to counter the effects of her slight curve. Next she upped her yoga classes to three times a week. Then, when she relocated to the Bay Area in the summer of her seventieth birthday, yoga became her mainstay. After five plus years of regular yoga practice, she says she's stronger now than when she started practicing regularly:

> As I approached seventy-one, I began to realize that the practices I was using were actually making me stronger! It is very clear that I have a stronger core and more flexibility. Now, instead of avoiding movements, I take them on! If there is a staircase, rather than an elevator, I take it. I try to turn invitations to meet for coffee or a meal into a time to walk, especially to walk the hills.[1]

Increasing your strength is ageless.

—Wayne Diamond, physical therapist and yoga teacher

And so far, in the past year, even with some periods of fatigue and stress, she rarely misses more than a few days of fairly vigorous yoga. She says, "My greatest joy comes when I can hold the balance and standing poses, especially Ardha Chandrasana and Vasisthasana and various supported inversions—my favorite challenge moves!"[2]

STRENGTH

Strength is the first of our four essential physical skills because we need muscle strength just to move through our daily lives—to get out of bed in the morning, stand up in the shower, get dressed, cook breakfast, and get in and out of the car. We need even more strength to stay physically active, whether that means hiking, cycling, playing sports, gardening, repairing the house, or playing with the grandkids, and for extended activity of any kind we need endurance as well as strength.

In addition, strong muscles help to protect your joints—your muscles take up some of the weight and pressure, so the joints are not doing all the work themselves. That's why, for example, if you have arthritis of the knees, working to maintain leg strength is so beneficial.

If we don't maintain our muscle strength as we age, muscular weakness can lead to an inability to live independently because even the simplest of daily activities, such as getting out of a chair or walking up or down the stairs, require strength. Muscular weakness can also compromise our ability to balance, increasing our risk of falling, which can cause broken bones or other serious injuries.

Then there are our bones. Although we tend to think of muscles alone as creating strength, our bones support our muscles and our muscles use our bones to move us through the world. So strong, healthy bones are an integral part of physical strength. In addition, it's important to keep bones strong so they don't break or fracture.

For healthy aging, muscle and bone strength are equally important! Before discussing how you can use yoga to foster their strength, let's have a look at how aging affects both.

Aging and Strength

Just as the natural aging process affects all organs, structures, and systems of your body, it also affects muscle and bone strength. Because both muscles and bones contribute to your overall strength, loss of strength in one is typically associated with loss in the other, so it's equally important to actively maintain muscle and bone strength. Fortunately, using yoga to maintain your muscle strength will help with bone strength and vice versa.

MUSCLES. We have more than 640 muscles in our bodies and starting as early as our thirties, these muscles gradually lose strength. This natural aging process, called skeletal muscle atrophy, causes your muscle cells and fibers to become smaller and weaker, leading to a loss of muscle mass, quality, and strength. The rate at which we lose muscle strength varies from person to person and is influenced by behavioral, genetic, and environmental factors.

Behavioral factors. How physically active you are overall influences how quickly you will lose muscle strength. If you have a sedentary job or lifestyle and do not exercise, you're going to lose strength more quickly than if your job or lifestyle is physically demanding or you exercise regularly. Your eating habits also influence your strength, as poor nutrition can worsen muscle atrophy.

Genetic factors. Your body type can influence how weak you become with age. If you tended to have larger muscles as a young adult, you simply have more muscle mass to lose as you age before you become weak. On the other hand, if you're someone who tended not to bulk up easily, you may become weaker more quickly as you age. Although you cannot change your body type, if you have not already started to do so, you can begin building up your muscles now as a preventative measure. Yoga's strength-building poses and techniques provide an excellent way to do this.

In general, men lose muscle mass at a slightly faster rate than women until women reach menopause, when the more rapid loss of bone that women experience (see below) contributes to greater loss of muscle strength as well. So leading up to and during menopause, women should focus especially on maintaining muscle strength.

Illnesses and injuries. Muscle disuse can accelerate loss of muscle strength. This disuse can be the result of joint injuries, arthritis, stroke, illnesses (such as diabetes, cancer, and HIV/AIDS) that affect the nerves and the blood supply to muscles as well as having other negative effects, and medications that weaken or damage muscles. For those who are dealing with these conditions, you can slow down the loss of strength by starting to move again with yoga.

Sarcopenia. A low percentage of people—whether due to illness, long-time inactivity, or just very advanced age—lose so much muscle mass that they reach an advanced stage of skeletal muscle atrophy called "sarcopenia." Sarcopenia is the disease stage of skeletal muscle atrophy, just as osteopenia and osteoporosis are two disease stages of age-related bone loss.

Naturally, this serious loss of muscle mass—which is accompanied by significant muscle weakness—is something you want to avoid if at all possible because serious muscle weakness is one of the main factors that can lead to loss of independence. Fortunately, gentle forms of yoga can help even very elderly and weak people regain strength.

BONES. We have 204 bones in our skeletons, and like our muscles, those bones undergo changes as we age, gradually becoming thinner and weaker. However, it is only when our bones reach a certain degree of thinness that we are at greater risk of a fracture from a fall or poor postural habits. The rate at which we lose bone strength varies from person to person and is also influenced by behavioral, genetic, and environmental factors.

Behavioral factors. The same behavioral factors that have a negative effect on muscle strength, such as a sedentary lifestyle and poor nutrition, contribute to bone loss as well. In addition, regular use of certain medications, including steroids in high doses, cancer drugs, and some heartburn medicines, can also contribute to bone loss.

Genetic factors. Your body type, race, ethnicity, and natural bone density can influence how weak your bones become with age. Some people just naturally have thinner and/or less dense bones, so they have less bone mass to lose before bones become weak and brittle. For women, hormonal changes during menopause or due to other reasons accelerate the rate of bone loss, which is why more women develop osteoporosis in their fifties. Although you cannot change your genes or gender, if you have not already started to do so, you can begin strengthening your bones now as a preventative measure.

OSTEOPOROSIS. While everyone's bones thin somewhat as they age, for some people, due to advanced age, illness, medications, or menopause for women, bone loss can reach a critical point, which is called "osteoporosis." At this stage, the bones are more vulnerable to fractures and are also slower to heal. (Osteopenia is the stage of bone loss just before full osteoporosis, when you are already starting to be at risk for fractures from falls but not to the same degree as osteoporosis.)

Both body type and gender influence how weak bones become with age. People with smaller bones are at greater risk of developing osteoporosis than those with larger bones. And women in general are at greater risk than men. However, for both men and women, developing osteoporosis is common, so it's wise for everyone to take precautions.

For those with osteoporosis, the bones of the thoracic spine (your mid-spine) are at the greatest risk for fracture, followed by the wrist bones and the thighbones at the hip joints. These fractures can lead to chronic pain, physical disability, and, particularly with hip fractures, premature death. Because yoga is weight bearing, it could reverse bone loss, and practicing yoga balance poses is very helpful for preventing falls, which are actually more responsible for causing fractures than osteoporosis.

How Yoga Helps

Because a balanced asana practice includes standing poses, backbends, forward bends, twists, and inverted poses, a regular practice that includes a wide range of poses will build strength in both muscles and bones throughout your entire body.

Muscle Strength and Endurance

To do any active yoga pose, you contract certain muscles to enter in and out of the pose as well as to hold it. Although this muscle contraction does not result in bulky muscles, it very effectively lengthens, tones, and strengthens your muscles. Improving your muscle strength with yoga not only allows you to hold your static poses longer, it also provides the strength you need for your everyday activities and other types of exercise. The sheer variety of poses ensures that you can strengthen all the important muscles in your body, and practicing for longer sessions helps increase endurance as well as strength.

Bone Strength

In your yoga asana practice, you take many weight-bearing positions on your feet, as well as on other parts of your body, such as your hands, sitting bones, and shins. All of these weight-bearing poses load your bones, which naturally builds bone strength. In addition, the muscle contractions you use to stay in a pose stimulate your bones to strengthen themselves more vigorously than weight bearing alone, and the great variety of poses means that you will be strengthening *all* of your bones.

Static and Dynamic Poses

Holding a static pose strengthens your muscles through isometric muscle contraction, and you can add in conscious muscle activation as described under "Muscle Activation" (see page 36) to enhance this. If you gradually increase how long you hold a pose over time, you will improve endurance as well as strength. Eventually you can hold poses for one or two minutes or even longer. If you are practicing for bone strength, we recommend holding a yoga pose for thirty seconds or more, as Dr. Loren Fishman's ten-year study on yoga for osteoporosis showed that this length of time can be effective for building bone strength.

Moving in and out of a dynamic pose strengthens you in a different way than staying in the full pose. As your muscles move you into and out of the pose, they are being strengthened through resistance training rather than isometric muscle contraction. In addition, they are being strengthened throughout a greater range of motion (in every step along the way into and out of the pose) rather than just in the shape of the full pose. So if you do a set of dynamic pose repetitions, you're working your muscles very differently than if you just hold the pose for the same length of time.

Although we don't know of any studies on dynamic poses and bone strength, we do know that normal movement, such as walking and running, strengthens bones. So it's likely that practicing a pose dynamically in sets of repetitions is going to strengthen bones as well as muscles.

You can see there are different benefits to each way of practicing. So generally it looks like doing some of both is the way to go, if you're up for it! You can either mix static and dynamic poses within a single practice or alternate them on different days.

USING YOGA FOR STRENGTH

All poses, except restorative poses, are weight bearing (even if you're bearing weight on some body part other than your feet), and all active poses require muscle contraction in some form, so any active yoga pose will strengthen both your bones and muscles. A well-rounded active yoga practice that includes a good mix of standing poses, backbends, twists, and forward bends will provide all-around muscle- and bone-strength building. But if you'd like to focus on strengthening a particular area, for example, if you have knee arthritis and want to work on leg strength, you can choose the corresponding categories shown in the table below to emphasize in your practice.

Leg and hip strength	Any poses where you stand on one or both legs, especially with one or both knees bent (e.g., Powerful Pose) or where you lift your leg or legs away from the ground (e.g., Locust Pose or Boat Pose), strengthen the legs and hips.
Arm and shoulder strength	Any pose where you bear weight on your hands (e.g., Downward-Facing Dog Pose) or forearms or where you lift your arms away from the floor, either out to the sides (Warrior 2 Pose), overhead (Warrior 1 Pose), or forward or behind your back (Locust Pose) will strengthen your arms and shoulders. To strengthen your wrists with yoga, you need to bear weight on your hands.
Core strength	Any poses where you lift your leg or legs away from the floor (e.g., Hunting Dog Pose, Locust Pose, and Boat Pose), tip your torso to the side (e.g., Triangle Pose), lift your hips away from the floor (e.g., Plank Pose, Side Plank Pose, or Upward Plank Pose), or activate your core muscles (e.g., Boat Pose, Hunting Dog Pose, and Plank Pose) strengthen your core.
Back and spinal strength	Standing and seated twists help strengthen spinal bones and the muscles of your back that support your spine. Standing, prone, and supine backbends strengthen overall back muscles.

Techniques for Building Muscle and Bone Strength

HOW LONG TO HOLD THE POSES. For muscle strength in static poses, you can work on either strength or endurance. To work on muscle strength alone, hold the pose for at least thirty seconds if possible and consider repeating the pose several times. To work on endurance, hold the pose as long as you safely can, gradually working up to longer holds of one to two minutes. For bone strength in static poses, we recommend holding the pose for thirty seconds or more.

If you're too weak or fatigued to stay in a pose for the recommended time, hold the pose for as long as you safely can and then come out. Gradually over the next several weeks, work your way up to longer and longer holds.

For muscle or bone strength in dynamic poses, move in and out of the pose with your breath for six or more repetitions.

HOW OFTEN TO DO THE POSES. When you are working on strength building, the muscles you're strengthening need a day of rest between exercise sessions. So generally you shouldn't exercise the same muscle group on consecutive days. However, you can do strength-building yoga poses every day if you focus on different areas of your body each day, for example, alternating between upper body, lower body, and core strength. Or, you can alternate strength-building practice days with gentle stretching, restorative yoga, or breath-work sessions and/or meditation. If you are practicing for bone strength, follow the same recommendations.

BALANCED PRACTICE. To balance your strength building, make sure your practice includes poses of all of the basic types—standing poses, backbends, forward bends, and twists—as long as these are safe for you. Of course you don't need to do all these basic types within a single practice; just try to get to them sometime each week. Also, try to include poses where you bear weight on your hands as well as on your sitting bones, shins, and so on, such as Downward-Facing Dog Pose, Side Plank Pose, Hunting Dog Pose, and Boat Pose.

STRETCHING. Because your body's response to stretching and strengthening is similar in promoting muscle growth, poses that you might think of as "just stretching" also enhance strength. So when you practice for flexibility (see chapter 4), you'll be increasing strength. You can also enhance your strength building in a stretch (and improve the stretch) by adding in muscle activation.

MUSCLE ACTIVATION. Although a weight-bearing pose on its own will strengthen the bones that are bearing your weight, the bone strengthening effect is enhanced by consciously contracting the muscles holding you up. Do this by gently firming your muscles toward the bones rather than contracting them so strongly that they bulge away from the bones. For example, if you're standing in Tree Pose, firming your leg muscles will enhance bone building in the standing leg.

You can strengthen more than just the obviously active muscles by consciously contracting other muscles as you work in the pose. For example, in Downward-Facing Dog Pose, firm all your arm and shoulder muscles toward the bones. When you want to strengthen your hip area, in a standing pose, for example, you can slowly engage the muscles all around your hip joints, as long as this action does not pull you out of good alignment.

The reason we're always encouraging you to contract your muscles gently by firming them toward the bone is because strongly contracting a muscle noticeably shortens the muscle, which seems to prevent you from moving as freely in the pose. On the other hand, gently firming a muscle toward the bone provides muscular support without interfering with movement. If you're not used to working this way, it may take some practice. Take it in two steps:

1. Consciously relax the muscle, allowing it to lengthen.
2. Gently firm the muscle toward the bone.

UPPER BODY STRENGTH PRACTICE

This sequence is designed to strengthen all of the muscles in your upper body, including the upper spine, shoulders, neck, and arms, by combining static and dynamic strength-building poses.

As you practice, focus on inviting a sense of strength and vitality into the muscles you feel working. To enhance the strength-building effects of the static poses, including Lunge Pose, Extended Side Angle Pose, and Warrior 2 Pose, try intentionally contracting your arm and shoulder muscles as you hold the pose. Between poses, if you notice your wrists are sore, shake out your hands and wrists for a few seconds. For information on practicing breath awareness, see "How to Practice Breath Awareness" in chapter 9.

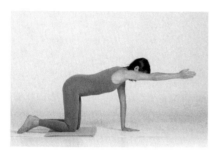

1. Hunting Dog Pose, version 3, 30–60 seconds each side

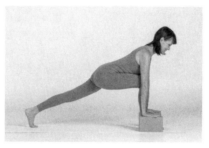

2. Lunge Pose, version 2 or 4, 30–60 seconds each side

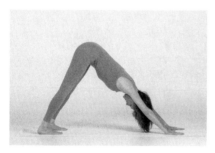

3. Downward-Facing Dog Pose, any version, 1–2 minutes

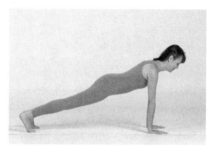

4. Plank Pose, version 1, 3, or 4, 30 seconds, 2 times

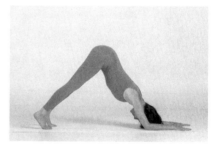

5. Downward-Facing Dog Pose, version 4, 30 seconds

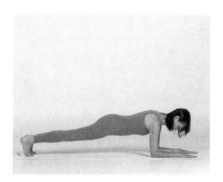

6. Plank Pose, version 2, 30 seconds

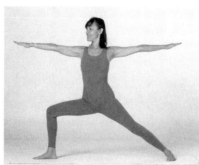

7. Warrior 2 Pose, version 1 or 3, 30–60 seconds each side

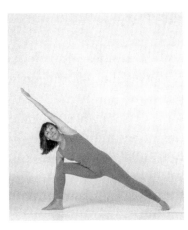
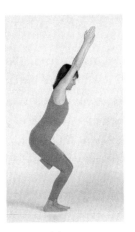
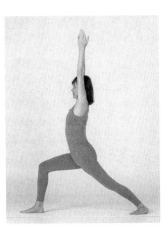
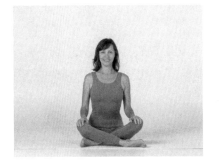

8. Extended Side Angle Pose, any version, 1–2 minutes each side

9. Powerful Pose, version 2, 30–60 seconds

10. Warrior 1 Pose, version 1 or 2, 1–2 minutes each side

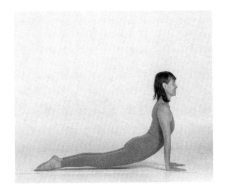
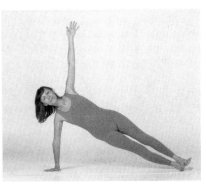
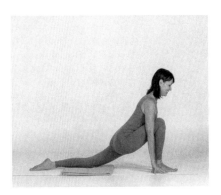

11. Upward-Facing Dog Pose, version 1, 2, or 3, 30 seconds

12. Side Plank Pose, any version, 30–60 seconds each side

13. Lunge Pose, version 4, 1 minute each side

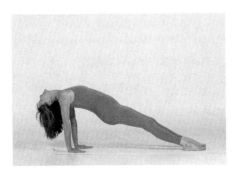
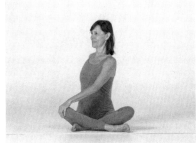
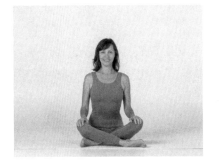

14. Upward Plank Pose, any version, 30–60 seconds

15. Easy Sitting Twist, any version, 30–60 seconds each side

16. Easy Sitting Pose, version 1, 2, or 3, 2–4 minutes, with breath awareness

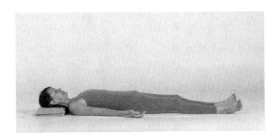

17. Relaxation Pose, version 2, 5–10 minutes

LOWER BODY STRENGTH PRACTICE

This sequence is designed to strengthen all of the muscles in your lower body, including your leg, hip, and lower back muscles, by combining static stretching poses with dynamic poses.

As you practice, focus on inviting a sense of strength and vitality into the areas where you feel your muscles working. To enhance the strength-building effects of the static poses, try intentionally contracting your leg and hip muscles as you hold the pose. In Lunge Pose, try keeping your fingertips only lightly on the ground or a block to encourage your legs and hip muscles to work harder.

For photos that illustrate the individual movements in the dynamic poses, see the "Dynamic Poses and Flow Sequences" section on page 282.

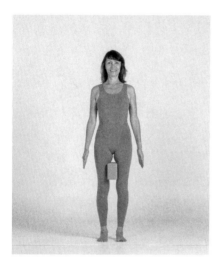

1. Mountain Pose, version 2, 1–2 minutes

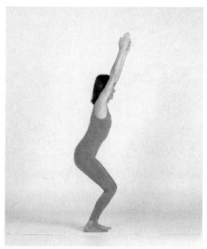

2. Dynamic Powerful Pose, 6 times

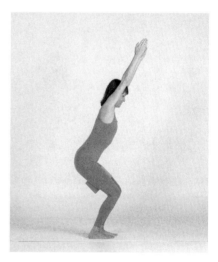

3. Powerful Pose, version 2, 30–60 seconds

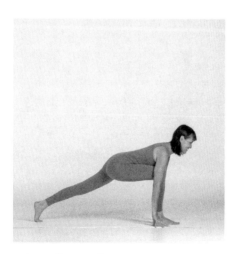

4. Lunge Pose, version 1, 2, or 3, 30–60 seconds each side

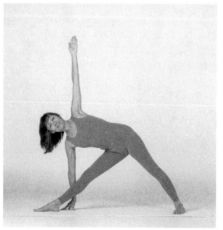

5. Triangle Pose, any version, 1–2 minutes each side

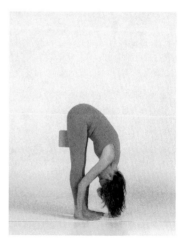

6. Standing Forward Bend, version 3, 1 minute

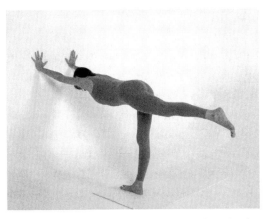

7. Warrior 3 Pose, version 2, 30–60 seconds each side

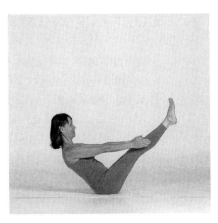

8. Boat Pose, any version, 30–60 seconds

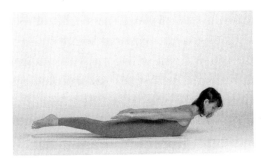

9. Dynamic Locust Pose, 6 times

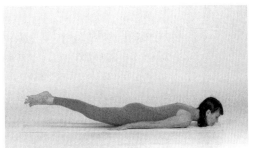

10. Locust Pose, version 4, up to 30 seconds

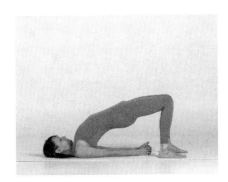

11. Bridge Pose, version 1, 30–90 seconds

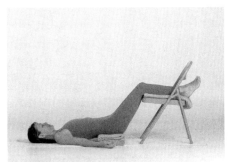

12. Legs Up the Wall Pose, version 4, 3–5 minutes

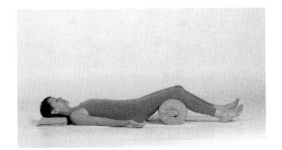

13. Relaxation Pose, version 3, 5–10 minutes

CORE STRENGTH PRACTICE

This sequence is designed to strengthen all of your core muscles, including your abdominal, lower back, and pelvic-floor muscles and your diaphragm. Dynamic Reclined Twist, Plank Pose, Boat Pose, Hunting Dog Pose, Extended Side Angle Pose, and Triangle Pose will strengthen your abdominal muscles. Cobra Pose, Dynamic Locust Pose, and Hunting Dog Pose will strengthen your lower back muscles. Plank Pose, Hunting Dog Pose, and Boat Pose will strengthen your pelvic-floor muscles and diaphragm. The sequence winds down with supported Reclined Cobbler's Pose to allow all your core muscles to relax.

As you practice the poses, focus on creating a sense of strength and stability throughout your entire core and maintain a steady breath. In Dynamic Reclined Twist, to increase the work of your abdominal muscles, try lightly resting your legs on the floor just for a moment before coming back up. For Triangle Pose and Extended Side Angle Pose, to provide more strengthening for your side abdominal muscles, try resting only your bottom hand lightly on the floor or a block.

For photos that illustrate the individual movements in the dynamic poses, see the "Dynamic Poses and Flow Sequences" section on page 282.

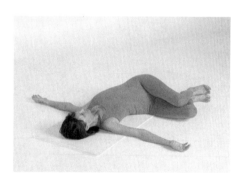

1. Dynamic Reclined Twist, 6 times

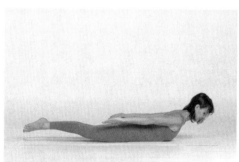

2. Dynamic Locust Pose, 6 times

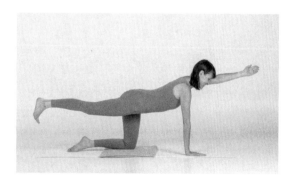

3. Hunting Dog Pose, version 1, 30–90 seconds each side

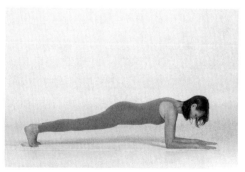

4. Plank Pose, version 2, 30–60 seconds

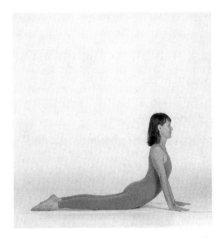

5. Cobra Pose, any version, 30–60 seconds

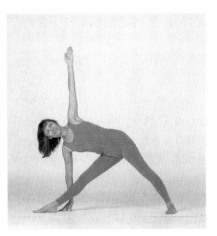

6. Triangle Pose, version 1, 2 or 3, 30 seconds each side

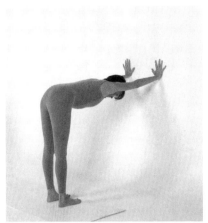

7. Half Downward-Facing Dog Pose, any version, 1 minute

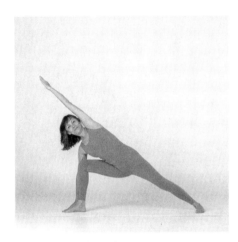

8. Extended Side Angle Pose, version 1, 2, or 3, 30 seconds each side

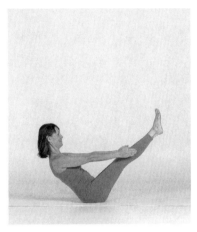

9. Boat Pose, any version, 30–60 seconds, 2 times

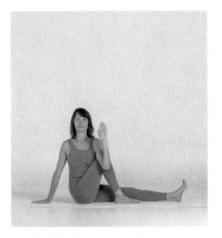

10. Sage's Twist 3, any version, 1 minute each side

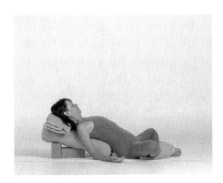

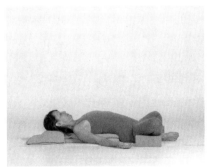

11. Reclined Cobbler's Pose, version 2 or 3, 5 minutes

BONE STRENGTH PRACTICE

This well-rounded sequence is designed to help you build bone strength in your most vulnerable bones. The practice includes weight-bearing poses on both your hands and feet, which build strength in your hips and wrists, and backbends, which target the bones of your spine.

To maximize bone building, hold the poses for the specified times if it's possible for you. In every pose, focus on intentionally activating as many muscles as you can. For example, in Warrior 1 Pose, intentionally firm the muscles all around your shoulder joints and the knee of your back leg. Because the first four poses require weight bearing on your hands and wrists, feel free to rest at any point between the poses to shake out your hands and wrists.

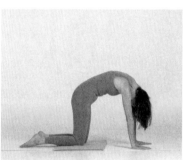

1. Dynamic Cat-Cow Pose, 6 times

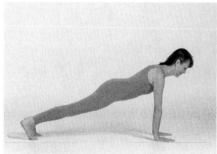

2. Hunting Dog Pose, version 1, 30–60 seconds each side

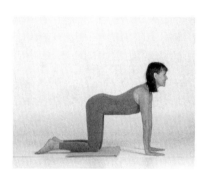

3. Downward-Facing Dog Pose, any version, 30–60 seconds

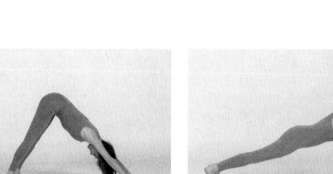

4. Plank Pose, any version, 30–60 seconds

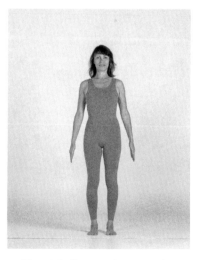

5. Mountain Pose, version 1, 1 minute

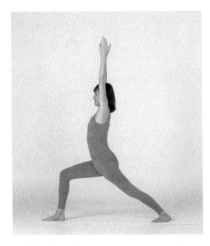

6. *Warrior 1 Pose, any version, 30–60 seconds each side*

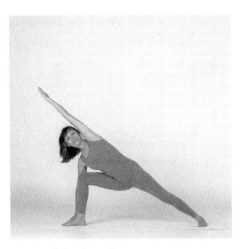

7. *Extended Side Angle Pose, any version, 30–60 seconds each side*

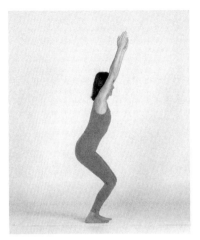

8. *Powerful Pose, any version, 30–60 seconds*

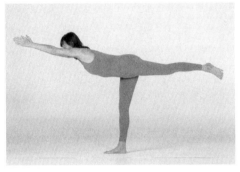

9. *Warrior 3 Pose, any version, 20–30 seconds each side*

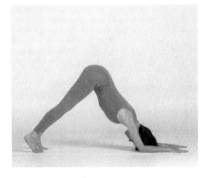

10. *Downward-Facing Dog Pose, version 4, 30 seconds*

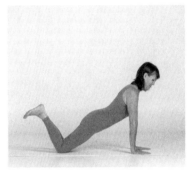

11. *Plank Pose, version 4, 30 seconds*

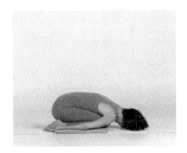

12. *Child's Pose, any version, 1 minute*

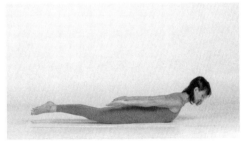

13. *Locust Pose, any version, 30 seconds, 2 times*

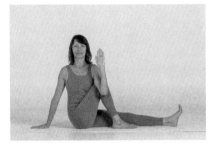

14. *Sage's Twist 3, any version, 30-60 seconds each side*

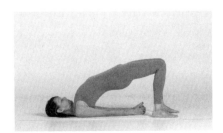

15. *Bridge Pose, version 1, 30 seconds, 2 times*

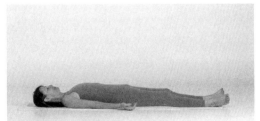

16. *Relaxation Pose, any version, 5 minutes*

4

Yoga for Flexibility

FLEXIBILITY IS THE SECOND OF OUR FOUR ESSENTIAL PHYSICAL skills because just as you need strength to move you through the world, you need flexibility to make all those movements. Several different muscles are stretched with every movement you make. For example, if you raise your arm in front of you and overhead with the palm facing up, the muscles and fascia on the underside of your arm and shoulder are stretching as you use your strength to do the actual lifting. Without those muscles and fascia stretching, your arm would just be stuck in place! So you can see why some amount of flexibility is necessary just to do the simplest physical tasks—get out of bed in the morning, wash your hair, dress yourself, cook breakfast, and walk down the street. And, of course, if you're going to stay physically active—whether that means taking care of your house by gardening and doing repairs, enjoying physical activities such as dancing and swimming, or just looking after small children—you need more than just basic flexibility. Flexibility is also an important element of balance, as responding to uneven surfaces or unexpected obstacles requires moving quickly and easily.

For many years, both of us have been working on flexibility for different reasons. Baxter focuses on flexibility because he's naturally very stiff. In fact, in his early days of yoga practice, when he would try to do a Standing Forward Bend with his knees straight, his hands wouldn't even make it to his knees, and the stretch felt quite intense! But, although it took some time and regular practice, after a couple of years, he noticed he was getting his fingers to the floor with minimal effort and was actually liking it. As his practice deepened, this process repeated itself in many areas of his body. He also noticed that being more flexible contributed to his sense of physical well-being—becoming more flexible can be like switching to looser, more comfortable clothing—and made many of his other activities, such as biking and playing the violin, easier.

Nina was diagnosed with mild arthritis of the hip joint nine years ago (likely a result of her mild scoliosis of the spine), so she focuses on maintaining the mobility of her hips by regularly doing poses that stretch the muscles around the joint, something that maintains the health of the joints as well as their mobility. There's been no further deterioration and so far no need for the hip replacement that one doctor claimed would be necessary.

ABOUT FLEXIBILITY

Although the word *flexibility* makes most people think about the ability of muscles to lengthen—like that superhero Plastic Man—flexibility is really much more than that. And because there are some aspects of flexibility that you can change and others that you should not even try to change, understanding a bit about flexibility will help you choose the most appropriate practices while keeping you safe.

Technically your flexibility is the range of movement you have around a particular joint. For example, a person who is flexible in their shoulder joints can raise their arms higher and take them back farther than someone who is tight in that area. The range of motion you have in a particular joint is determined by the following:

- Size and shape of the bones that make up the joint
- Mechanics of that particular joint
- Condition of the tendons and ligaments attached to the joint
- Extensibility of the fascia as well as the muscles that move the joint

Let's look at each of these features separately, so you can understand what you can and cannot change and why.

Joints

Some joints have a greater range of motion than others because of the size and shape of the bones that they connect and the way the bones are connected. For example, your shoulder joint is a ball and socket that allows your arm bone to have a large range of motion, including moving out to the side or across your body, as well as overhead, behind your back, and rotating in the joint. Try it! Your knee joint, on the other hand, joins straight leg bones together in a hinge joint and restricts your movement to bending and straightening. Try bending and straightening your knees and then imagine making the other movements you did with your arms. You can see that your shoulder joint is inherently more flexible than your knee joint, and this is a condition you can't change.

In addition, because each joint has a complex structure in which several different components come together—bones, cartilage, tendons, joint capsule, synovial fluid, and so on—there can be great variation in the natural mobility of different people. For example, someone may have a unique skeletal structure that limits hip flexibility. These variations are beyond our control—all the stretching in the world will not change the structure of our joints.

Other factors that can affect the range of motion in your joints include injuries, such as meniscal tears in the knee joint, or health conditions that limit joint mobility, such as arthritis. While you cannot change many of these conditions, there are some, such as meniscal tears, that you can get medical care for and others, such as osteoarthritis, that you can improve with yoga.

Muscles and Fascia

Whenever you do a stretching movement, such as stretching your hamstring muscles (backs of your thighs) in Standing Forward Bend, you are lengthening those muscles. This action has a temporary effect on your muscles, but after you stop the action, your muscles will return to their resting length (their original size). However, with continued practice, you can make longer-lasting changes in a muscle, so that its resting length is longer. This is one way we can change our bodies with yoga, becoming more flexible over time with ongoing practice.

When you stretch a muscle, you are also stretching the fascia that surrounds and supports the muscle. Fascia is a specialized tissue that surrounds all organs, muscles, and individual muscle fibers in the body as well as bones, blood vessels, and nerves, and it is the layer of tissue immediately under your skin. Like muscles, fascia can change in length, both temporarily and permanently. But because its makeup is different from a muscle's, it takes longer to change the resting length of fascia than it does to change the resting length of muscles.

In addition to supporting individual muscles, fascia forms planes that run long distances through your body. Like muscles, these planes of fascia can become tight and restricted. For example, there is a plane of fascia that runs from the tops of your feet up to the front of your throat. Years of poor posture (with forward rounding) can make this plane of fascia tight, restricting your ability to sit or stand up straight.

So when you are working on flexibility, it's a good idea to address your fascia as well as your muscles by stretching your entire body—either front, side, or back—rather than isolated areas. For example, to address the tightness in the plane of fascia restricting your ability to stand up straight, you could practice Mountain Pose and supported backbends.

Tendons and Ligaments

A tendon is a tough tissue that connects a muscle to a bone. This connective tissue is the continuation of fascia that attaches the muscle it surrounds to a bone. For example, a thick tendon connects your hamstring muscles to your lower leg bone (you can easily feel this one at the back of your outer knee).

However, because a tendon is made of strong connective tissue, it is inherently less stretchy than fascia or muscles, so you should never try to stretch tendons. If you do, you risk tearing the tendons, which can cause inflammation—painful!

Ligaments keep two adjacent bones close together to provide stability for the joint, while allowing some movement at the joint. For example, the ligaments in your knee joint determine how far you can take your lower leg bones in each direction. Ligaments are made of connective tissue similar to that of tendons, and like tendons, you should never try to stretch ligaments because it can tear them and injure the joint.

So if you feel a stretching sensation near a joint, such as a knee, hip, shoulder, or elbow joint, back off immediately from the stretch. If that doesn't help, come out of the pose.

Variability

Anyone observing us practicing Standing Forward Bend would immediately see that even though we're both longtime practitioners, our ability to stretch the muscles in the backs of our legs varies greatly. Nina can get her hands flat on the ground, while Baxter can only touch his fingertips to the floor. Yes, it turns out that flexibility among people varies and often quite a bit! Some people are naturally tight, some are naturally flexible, and others are overly flexible.

There are three factors that influence our flexibility:

1. Amount of flexibility in the stabilizing structures of the joint capsule and ligaments—You might detect this by sensing restrictions near your joints.

2. Muscle length or fascial tightness—You might detect this by sensing restriction midmuscle or along the length of a muscle group.

3. Diseases that affect flexibility—Certain common diseases, such as arthritis or Parkinson's disease, can gradually reduce flexibility over time. Other rare conditions can have more extreme effects on flexibility, such as Ehlers-Danlos syndrome, which makes people hypermobile, and scleroderma, which severely restricts people. In addition, certain medical conditions can temporarily limit flexibility in specific areas, such as frozen shoulder or acute shoulder bursitis, which would limit the movement of the shoulder joint.

Although there is no official standard for "average flexibility," you can assess yourself by doing the following basic poses and comparing your range of motion and flexibility to those of fellow practitioners, or by having your teacher watch you do them and give you feedback on where you fall on the flexibility scale:

- Standing Forward Bend
- Crescent Moon variation of Arms Overhead Pose
- Triangle Pose
- Lunge Pose
- Bridge Pose
- Cobbler's Pose
- Easy Sitting Twist

Be aware, however, that flexibility can vary quite a bit from joint to joint. For example, you might be flexible in the shoulders but tight in the hips. So be careful not to label yourself as stiff or flexible without a good examination of your flexibility in all areas of your body.

Once you have identified your tight areas, you might want to focus your attention on increasing flexibility in those areas. For example, if you are particularly tight in the hamstrings, it makes sense to emphasize leg stretches.

So, when thinking about how to practice yoga for flexibility, be sure to take a good look at your body as well as your health history. This will enable you to design a customized practice that will benefit you as an individual and help keep you safe.

Before discussing how you can use yoga to foster flexibility, let's have a look at how aging affects this essential physical skill.

Aging and Flexibility

You may not notice a gradual loss of flexibility until, say, the first day in early spring that you start to work in your garden and you realize it's a bit harder than it used it be and maybe even painful. Yes, as we age, our flexibility slowly decreases. Although some of this is due to age-related changes, a sedentary lifestyle can accelerate the process. Because several factors influence your flexibility, let's take a closer look at how aging affects each of those factors and which of them you can influence with your yoga practice.

MUSCLES. As you age, your muscles and the individual fibers within them gradually shrink and lose mass, and you actually lose some of the muscle fibers. In addition to these age-related changes, muscles can shrink and tighten over time due to behavioral and environmental factors, such as inactivity or habitual ways of standing and sitting. This overall shrinking of your muscles means that they literally cannot stretch as far as they did when you were younger.

In addition, as you age, your muscles take longer to respond to stretching exercises than they did when you were young. So you may have to work more patiently to achieve improvements. However, practicing a wide variety of stretching poses can help you maintain the flexibility and health of your muscles.

FASCIA. The connective tissue that surrounds every muscle in your body tends to gradually dry out and become more inflexible with age. In addition, your fascia, like your muscles, can shrink and tighten because of behavioral and environmental factors, such as inactivity or habitual ways of standing and sitting. Practicing a wide variety of stretching poses will help you maintain the flexibility and health of your fascia as well as your muscles.

TENDONS AND LIGAMENTS. As you age, the water content of both tendons and ligaments gradually decreases, making the tissues stiffer. This will restrict the range of motion in your joints and lead to an overall decrease in flexibility. While you should not actively stretch your tendons or ligaments (this could damage them!), regularly stretching your muscles and fascia will indirectly benefit your tendons and ligaments by bringing nourishment to them and the joints they are connected to.

JOINTS. As some people age, the cartilage within their joints can gradually break down, causing inflammation in the joint, or osteoarthritis.

This inflammation reduces the range of motion in the joint because fluid buildup makes movement more painful and restricted. You can reduce the pain and swelling of arthritic joints and increase movement by practicing non-weight-bearing movements in appropriate yoga poses. Depending on your current condition, with continued practice, you may even be able to return to normal movement.

How Yoga Helps

Although yoga certainly isn't "just stretching," as some people think, yoga is definitely very effective for increasing flexibility. The huge variety of yoga poses allows you to stretch virtually all of your muscles. Some of those poses, such as Reclined Leg Stretch, are obvious "stretching" poses. But really just about every single pose except Relaxation Pose is automatically stretching at least some of your muscles. Even a pose that you may think of as primarily strengthening, such as Warrior 1 Pose, is stretching your front and back hips, your chest, and your shoulder joints. So just doing a well-rounded yoga practice that includes standing poses, backbends, forward bends, and twists will help you maintain flexibility.

Range of Motion

The vast array of yoga poses also allows you to move your joints in every direction, taking them through their entire range of motion. For example, the Reclined Leg Stretch series takes your hip joint forward, to the side, and across your body. Add in Lunge Pose, which takes the hip of your back leg behind you, and you've covered all four hip movements. In many other types of exercise, such as walking, running, and cycling, you simply repeat the same movements over and over. Although they provide cardiovascular and strength benefits, they don't improve your range of motion and can actually make you less flexible over time.

Moving your joints through their full range of motion with yoga—something you wouldn't be doing in your everyday life—also helps keep your joints healthy. The movements massage your joints, improving the flow of vital nutrition to them, which helps keep arthritis at bay.

Although you might not get to every single joint in a given day, if you vary your practice—something we highly recommend—by the end of the week you will have gotten around to all of them!

Fascia

Full body shapes that you hold for extended periods, such as Warrior 1 Pose and Standing Forward Bend, stretch your fascia as well as individual muscles. In particular, the various standing poses, especially those with feet wide apart, stretch your entire body, from feet to fingertips. Certain supported poses, such as Supported Backbend and Supported Standing Forward Bend, provide a good, long stretch for your fascial planes.

Props and Supported Poses

Of course many people start out with a limited range of motion, whether it's due to natural stiffness, injury, or illness. But by using props, you can do at least some version of almost every pose, which enables you to move each joint in the full range that's available to you. And when you become more flexible, you can gradually reduce or even eliminate your use of a prop.

Props also allow you to stay in a pose long enough to reap the full benefits (see the following section). And practicing fully supported poses, such as Supported Backbend and Supported Child's Pose, allows you to hold stretches for even longer periods (three to five minutes or longer) and to relax completely into the stretch. In the early days of her practice, Nina opened her chest, which was tight from years of sitting in front of a computer, by practicing Supported Backbend several times a week.

Dynamic vs. Static Poses

Practicing a pose dynamically or doing a short hold of a static pose can warm up your joints and make it easier to stretch your muscles during a given yoga practice, but it won't create lasting changes in your flexibility. In a day or two, your muscle will return to its resting length—the same length it was before you stretched it. However, recent research shows that when you hold a stretch for ninety seconds or more, the muscle protein titin changes shape, which can help a stretch last for several days. In addition, slow, gradual, longer stretches address tightness in fascia as well as in muscles. This means the type of stretching or flexibility practices you do depends on your goals.

STATIC POSES. Holding a static pose for more than twenty seconds is important because initially your muscle responds to being stretched with a protective contraction, and it only starts to relax and stretch after twenty seconds. So to warm up (that is, to create temporary flexibility that will enhance the rest of your practice), hold a static pose for thirty to ninety seconds. For example, you could warm up for standing poses by doing Reclined Leg Stretch variations for thirty seconds each. To create longer-lasting flexibility in both muscles and fascia, hold static poses for ninety seconds or more. If that seems like too much and you want to work on long-lasting flexibility, in many cases, you can use supported poses, such as Supported Child's Pose, to stretch the muscles. With any static pose, except supported poses, you can also add in muscle activation (see "Activating Muscles" on page 57) to enhance the stretch.

DYNAMIC POSES. Use slow, dynamic movements in and out of poses to create gradual muscle lengthening without triggering the protective reflex. These poses are a good way to warm up your joints in an easy fashion and can lead to immediate improvements in muscle flexibility, which you can then further with a static version of the same pose. For example, you could practice Dynamic Standing Forward Bend (see "Dynamic Poses and Flow Sequences" on page 282) to temporarily improve hamstring/hip flexibility, which you can then increase by holding the pose for ninety seconds. In general, we recommend practicing a combination of dynamic stretches for six to eight repetitions, followed by holding the static stretch for ninety seconds.

USING YOGA FOR FLEXIBILITY

Before you start to practice yoga for flexibility, consider how flexible you already are. If you're naturally tight or moderately flexible, working on flexibility either to improve or maintain it will be beneficial. You can use all the techniques we recommend for increasing resting muscle length and improving your range of motion, including both long holds and dynamic poses.

However, if you are overly flexible, practicing to become more flexible may actually be dangerous, as you risk worsening the lax support your joints already have. So even though being more flexible would enable you to do super bendy poses with greater ease, we recommend that you focus on strength instead. Include more strengthening poses in your practice and activate the muscles around your joints in all of your poses (see "Activating Muscles" on page 57)—even stretching poses—and always stretch less intensely.

Techniques for Improving and Maintaining Flexibility

HOW FAR TO STRETCH. When you stretch, be mindful not to go beyond the sensation of a healthy stretch into feelings of pain, burning, or compression in your joint (see "Healthy and Unhealthy Stretching Sensations" on page 58). If you experience sensations that feel unhealthy, either back off the stretch or use a prop or a different version of the pose. Overly flexible people should be extra careful, aiming for a lighter feeling of stretch or even doing the pose for strength instead flexibility by actively contracting their muscles instead of allowing them to stretch.

HOW LONG TO STRETCH. To cultivate long-lasting flexibility in your muscles and fascia, aim for holding a pose for at least ninety seconds. If this isn't possible, it might indicate that you are (1) stretching your muscle too far or that the opposing muscles are contracting too strongly, (2) the initial intensity of your stretch set off a strong protective reflex, or (3) you are doing a pose or a version of a pose that is too challenging for you. So start by backing off the stretch a bit or modifying the pose. If you just can't get comfortable, hold the pose until you are fatigued and gradually over time work your way up to longer holds.

Holding static poses for shorter periods will release the overnight tightness that we all experience and create temporary flexibility that will enhance the rest of your practice. For example, you could warm up for standing poses by doing leg stretches. Hold these warm-up stretches for at least thirty seconds to overcome the initial protective reflex.

HOW OFTEN TO STRETCH. To cultivate lasting flexibility, stretch a particular muscle or muscle group regularly, at least three times a week and at most every other day. In general, with consistent practice, you can see results for muscles after three to eight weeks. For fascia, however, it takes longer to create lasting changes—usually from three to six months.

You need to give your muscles a day of rest in between stretching sessions or you could develop an overuse injury. So generally you shouldn't stretch the same muscle group on consecutive days. However, you can do flexibility poses every day if you focus on different areas of your body; for example, alternating between upper body and lower body or between backbends and forward bends. Or, you can alternate intense stretching days with other types of yoga practice, such as active strength, balance, or agility practices, a gentle or restorative practice, or a pranayama/meditation practice on your off days.

STATIC POSES. Enter your static stretches slowly to allow your muscles to relax, release, and lengthen rather than tighten up. After you're in the pose, you can add in muscle activation on the opposite side of the joint to enhance the stretch (see "Activating Muscles" below).

DYNAMIC POSES. Practice dynamic poses at the beginning of your practice to warm up your joints and make the rest of your practice more comfortable. You can also practice the dynamic version of a pose as a way to warm up for the static version of the pose. For example, practice Bridge Pose dynamically to prepare for practicing the static version.

RESTORATIVE POSES. Practicing poses in which you relax as you gently stretch your body in a supported position are excellent for improving flexibility. For example, holding Supported Backbend for at least ninety seconds allows you to gently open your front body and holding Supported Child's pose for at least ninety seconds allows you to gently stretch your back body. Because planes of fascia run for long distances through your body, using a supported pose that stretches your entire body (front, side, or back) will stretch tight fascia as well as muscles.

BALANCE YOUR PRACTICE. To balance your flexibility practice, make sure it includes poses of all the basic types: standing poses, seated hip openers, backbends, forward bends, and twists, as long as these are safe for you. Of course you don't need to do all these basic types within a single practice; just try to do them sometime each week.

ACTIVATING MUSCLES. In static stretches, intentionally contracting the muscles on the opposite side of the joint—known as reciprocal inhibition—allows the muscle group you are stretching to lengthen more. So when you are stretching a particular muscle, bring your awareness to the antagonist muscle (the muscle opposite the one you are stretching) and gently activate it. For example, when stretching the front thigh muscles of your back leg in Lunge Pose, try consciously activating the back of your thigh. If you're not used to working this way, it may take some practice. Take it in two steps:

1. Consciously relax the muscle, allowing it to lengthen.
2. Gently firm the muscle toward the bone.

PROTECTING YOUR JOINTS. For people with joint problems, such as arthritis, consciously firming the muscles that support a problem joint will help protect the joint from strain or wear and tear. For example, if you have knee arthritis and are practicing Reclined Leg Stretch, you could firm the muscles around your knee joint as you bring your top leg into the pose and try to maintain that firmness as you stretch the back of your thigh.

For people who are overly flexible and can bend easily into deep forward bends and backbends, consciously activating the muscles that are supporting you in the pose will prevent you from hyperextending the joints. For example, in Standing Forward Bend, you can protect your hip joints by activating the muscles around the joints before you enter the pose and maintain as much of that as you can as you come into the pose. While the result will be a stretch that is not as deep as usual, your hip joints will benefit.

Overstretching can cause joint problems in supported poses as well as active poses. So if you feel any sensations of overstretching, pain, pinching, or compression while you are in a supported pose, come out of it and add more support to reduce the stretch. Likewise, if you notice pain in your joints after practicing supported poses, add more support the next time you practice.

Healthy and Unhealthy Stretching Sensations

Have you ever heard someone groaning in a yoga class? Or was that you? When you are stretching a tight area of your body, you can experience quite a bit of sensation. And while a healthy stretch can provoke an intense feeling, it's a good idea to pay attention to the type of sensation you're experiencing because this could indicate that you should back off the stretch.

As we discussed above, stretching a muscle or muscle group and fascia is healthy and beneficial, but stretching a tendon or ligament can cause an injury, such as a tear, inflammation, tendinitis, or tendinosis. In addition, compressing a joint when you are stretching can pinch the tissues caught between the bones moving toward each other, which causes pain and leads to inflammation. So it's important to learn to tell the difference between the sensation of a healthy stretch of a tight muscle versus the pain, pinching, or "smashed together" feelings that are warnings of potential injury.

HEALTHY SENSATIONS. You will generally feel a healthy muscle stretch toward the middle of a muscle, away from the tendons and ligaments that are located close to the joints. A good place to become familiar with this type of sensation is the hamstring muscles at the backs of your thighs which you stretch in Standing Forward Bend and Reclined Leg Stretch. As you may know, the intensity of the stretch sensation there can be quite strong, and yet it generally doesn't mean you are injuring yourself. So when you experience this type of sensation, as long as the stretch is a moderate one and in the middle of a muscle, take a deep breath and try to relax into the stretch.

UNHEALTHY SENSATIONS. You will generally feel an unhealthy stretch of muscle, tendon, or ligaments closer to a joint, such as your hip, knee, shoulder, or elbow joint. The quality of feeling will be different from that of a healthy stretch—maybe sharp, burning, stabbing, throbbing, or tearing in quality. For example, with the hamstring muscles, if you feel a tender burning sensation up toward your buttocks, this could indicate that you are overstretching the attachments. In all cases, when you experience these types of sensations, you should immediately back off the stretch to see if that helps. If not, come out of the pose entirely.

It is also possible to feel this sharp, burning, stabbing, throbbing, or tearing sensation in the muscle body as a result of a sudden, intense, quick stretch, so that is why we recommend always moving slowly and with control.

JOINT COMPRESSION. Sometimes when you are stretching a muscle, the joint that is bending can become compressed. For example, when you deeply bend your knee joints, as in Child's Pose, the tissues at the back of the knee joint can become pinched together. This is potentially dangerous because this compression could produce tissue damage and inflammation or could even injure nerves or blood vessels, leading to acute or chronic pain and dysfunction.

In general what you'll feel when a joint is compressed is either a pinching sensation or the feeling of muscles, skin, tendons, fascia, and/or bones being smashed together. For example, some less flexible practitioners feel smashed or pinching sensations in their front hip when doing Extended Side Angle Pose with their hand on the floor. Both of these sensations indicate that you are overdoing it, and you should back off the stretch, possibly by adding a prop. If you can't eliminate the joint compression, come out of the pose.

Compression can also put pressure on blood vessels and nerves, so if you have an unusual pressure sensation in the joint or feel numbness and tingling downstream from the compressed area, this also indicates that you are overdoing it and should back off the stretch or come out of the pose.

UPPER BODY FLEXIBILITY PRACTICE

This sequence is designed to improve upper body flexibility by including poses that stretch the muscles and fascia in your torso, shoulders, arms, and spine and move your shoulder joints through their entire range of motion. To improve your long-term flexibility, work on holding poses for longer periods of time, gradually progressing from the minimum time we specify to the maximum.

As you practice, focus on inviting a sense of release and lengthening wherever you experience a stretching sensation. In poses where your arms are actively stretching, such as Downward-Facing Dog, Arms Overhead, and Warrior 2 Pose, focus on lengthening your arms. In version 4 of Mountain Pose, remember to change the clasp of your hands and repeat the pose.

For photos that illustrate the individual movements in Dynamic Bridge Pose and Dynamic Warrior 1 Pose, see "Dynamic Poses and Flow Sequences" on page 282.

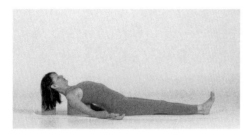

1. Supported Backbend, version 4, 1–3 minutes

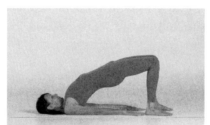

2. Dynamic Bridge Pose, 6 times

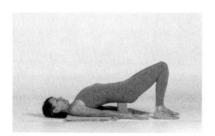

3. Bridge Pose, version 2 or 3, 1–3 minutes

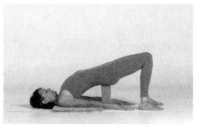

4. Downward-Facing Dog Pose, any version, 30–60 seconds

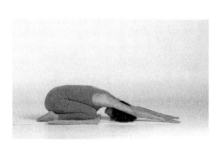

5. Child's Pose, version 2, 1–2 minutes

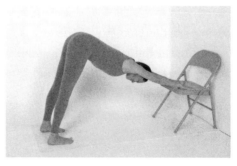

6. Downward-Facing Dog Pose, version 3, 30–60 seconds

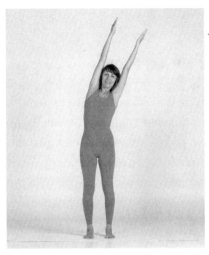

7. Arms Overhead Pose, version 4,
30–90 seconds to each side

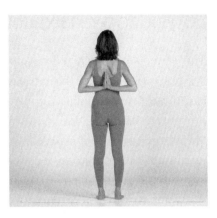

8. Mountain Pose, version 3 or 4, 30–90 seconds

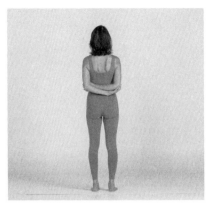

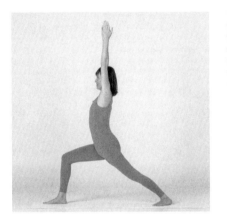

9. Dynamic Warrior 1 Pose, 6 times
each side

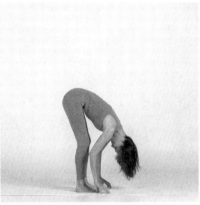

10. Standing Forward Bend, version 2,
1–2 minutes

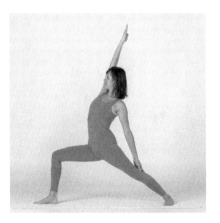

11. Warrior 2 Pose, version 4, 30–60
seconds each side

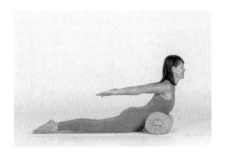

12. Locust Pose, version 2, 30–60 seconds

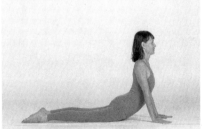

13. Cobra Pose, any version, 1–2 minutes

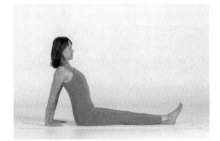

14. Upward Plank Pose, version 2,
30–90 seconds

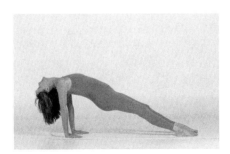

15. Upward Plank Pose, any version,
30–60 seconds

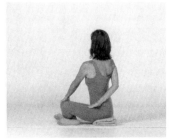

16. Easy Sitting Twist, version 2,
1–2 minutes each side

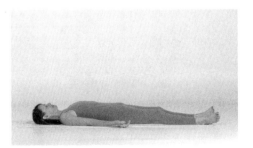

17. Relaxation Pose, any version, 5–10 minutes

LOWER BODY FLEXIBILITY PRACTICE

This sequence is designed to improve lower body flexibility by including poses that stretch the muscles in your legs, hips, and lower spine and move your hip joints through their entire range of motion. To improve your long-term flexibility, work on holding poses for longer periods of time, gradually progressing from the minimum time we specify to the maximum. As you practice, focus on relaxing and lengthening the muscles where you feel stretching sensations.

For instructions on practicing breath awareness, see "How to Practice Breath Awareness" on page 146.

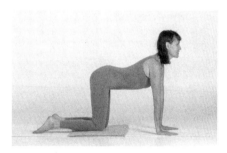

1. Reclined Twist, version 2, 1–2 minutes each side

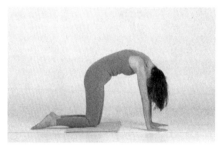

2. Reclined Leg Stretch, all 4 versions, 30–90 seconds each on each side

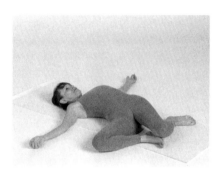

3. Dynamic Cat-Cow Pose, 6 times

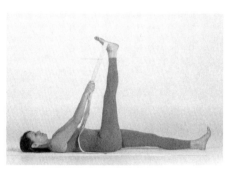

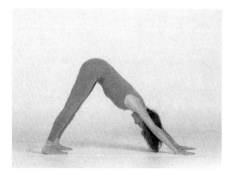

4. Mountain Pose, any version, 1 minute

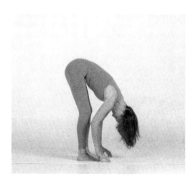

5. Standing Forward Bend, version 2, 30 seconds– 2 minutes

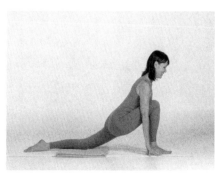

6. Lunge Pose, version 4, 1–2 minutes each side

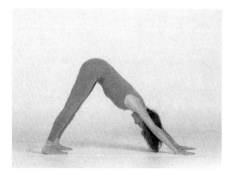

7. Downward-Facing Dog Pose, any version, 30–90 seconds

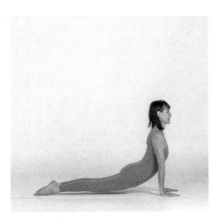

8. Upward-Facing Dog Pose, any version, 30–60 seconds

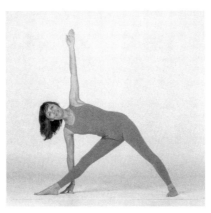

9. Triangle Pose, any version, 30–90 seconds each side

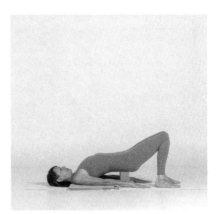

10. Bridge Pose, version 2, 3, or 4, 30 seconds–2 minutes

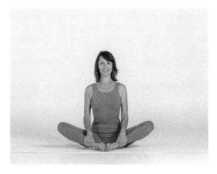

11. Cobbler's Pose, version 1, 2, or 3, 1–2 minutes

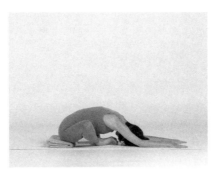

12. Cobbler's Pose, version 4, 30 seconds–2 minutes

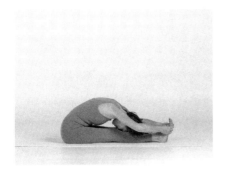

13. Seated Forward Bend, version 1 or 2, 1–2 minutes

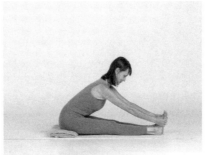

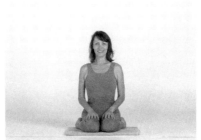

14. Child's Pose, any version, 2 minutes

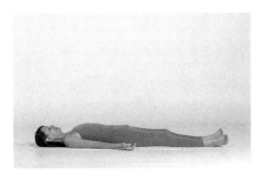

15. Relaxation Pose, any version, 5–10 minutes

16. Hero Pose, any version, 2–5 minutes, breath awareness

Yoga for Balance

FOR MOST OF HER ADULT LIFE, ANITA WAS "THE STRIDER"—
she regularly walked for miles with such a strong and confident stride that
she could run up three flights of stairs without a break. She was also relatively flexible and pretty much fearless. Then a few years ago as she was
striding down the street, she twisted her ankle on a piece of gravel and hit
the sidewalk hard, banging up her left knee and hip and wrenching her
back. By the time she had healed, she was very stiff—and she'd gotten
used to a very sedentary lifestyle. As she says, "Walking was more of a
shuffle and walking two blocks felt like a mile." She eventually did start
walking again, little by little, but a second fall on some winter ice completely "evaporated" every tiny bit of confidence she had built up. After
that, her fear of falling again made her withdraw from all physical activity,
and she was basically housebound. She says, "I thought I was at the end of
my healthy life, with a rigid body and a terrified mind."

That's when she reached out to us. We recommended three different
sequences for Anita to practice: a basic well-rounded sequence for improving strength, flexibility, and balance, a back-care practice, and a stress
management practice. Nina also recommended that Anita spend as much
time as possible barefoot.

This program helped Anita recover both her physical abilities and her
confidence. She says:

The moment I started practicing, I knew that I had the tools to positively effect a change and that translated, almost immediately, into regaining my confidence. And once I got my flexibility back, it was as if there was a mind-body reconnection as well. Although I sometimes backslide, when I do attend to the poses and sync my mind with my body, I feel pretty much invincible![1]

Balance is the ability to maintain a stable position. It is our third essential physical skill, because regardless of your age, maintaining your ability to balance is essential for safely going about your daily life. After all, you need to keep your balance when you're grabbing that bottle of peppercorns from the top shelf, carrying the basket of clean laundry up the stairs, or bending over to weed the tomato plants. Besides allowing you to maintain your independence, maintaining your ability to balance also allows you to continue participating in many of the activities that you love or that add richness to your life, such as spending time out in nature or traveling. And, of course, the ability to balance also helps prevent falls, which can be a serious—sometimes life-threatening—problem for older people.

Our ability to balance is actually surprisingly complex. Your brain takes in information from various systems in your body to determine how to move you back into balance. You also have postural reflexes that automatically kick in to keep you upright. But even when all balance systems and postural reflexes are functioning perfectly, your body won't be able to respond well to the information it's receiving from your brain if you're very weak or stiff. So maintaining strength, flexibility, and agility are key for maintaining your ability to balance. Maintaining your ability to focus mentally in the face of distraction is also essential because in the real world there's a lot going on all around us.

About Balance

Because understanding what influences your ability to balance will help you see what you can and cannot improve with yoga, let's take a closer look at how your brain gets the information it needs to keep you balanced. ("How Yoga Helps" on page 7 describes which of these factors you can improve with yoga.)

Vestibular System

The three canals in your inner ears provide your brain with information about changes in the position of your head, triggering reflexes that allow your body to maintain a steady posture. For example, from your head position, your vestibular system can tell if you're beginning to twist or spin or if you suddenly lurch forward, and it alerts your brain so you can self-correct. It also tells your brain if you're standing with your feet at different levels, such as when you're climbing up a rocky path or navigating a set of stairs.

Somatosensory System

Your senses provide your brain with information about the environment outside of your body, so you know where and how to move. For example, if you are walking outside, are you walking on solid ground or sinking into mud? Your senses include vision, touch, hearing, taste, and smell as well as proprioception (see page 7).

Visual System

Your eyes provide your brain with information about the position of your body relative to other objects in your environment, including their depth, velocity, and motion. You use this information to orient yourself. For example, when you're outside, you use the horizon to tell what "upright" is and when you're inside, you use the angles of the room in which you're standing to do the same. If you have poor eyesight, have you noticed what happens to your ability to balance when you're not wearing your glasses or contacts? Or have you ever closed your eyes in Tree Pose?

Touch

The sensors on your skin allow you to feel the outside environment. For example, your feet take in information about the type of surface you're walking or balancing on. And even if you're not on your feet, whatever part of your body is in contact with the ground provides feedback about the ground. For example, if you're balancing on one knee and one hand in Hunting Dog Pose, you'll feel the difference between practicing on the floor versus a stack of blankets. Touch also allows you to feel the environment around you, whether it's a strong wind pushing you slightly off balance or a wall that you're touching for support.

Proprioception

Sensors in all of your muscles and joints allow your brain to feel from the inside how your body is positioned, how it is moving through space, and where your body parts are relative to each other. The classic test for this is to close your eyes and then use your hand to touch your nose. In fact, proprioception is what allows you to walk around in the dark. When you're balancing, your proprioceptors tell your brain where your body is in the space so you know how to make adjustments to move back into balance.

Postural Reflexes

These reflexes automatically correct the orientation of your body when it shifts from being upright. They kick into action when unexpected events throw you off balance to try to prevent you from falling. Imagine turning and almost (or actually) bumping into someone, walking down a slick ramp and suddenly slipping, or reaching a crack in the sidewalk that trips you up. These reflexes also kick into action during everyday balancing activities, such as when you are getting dressed, standing on a chair in the kitchen to reach the upper shelf, or walking on the raised edge of a curb just for the fun of it.

Fortunately, yoga is particularly good at helping you maintain and even improve your ability to balance. But before discussing how you can use yoga to improve your balance, let's have a look at how aging affects this essential physical skill.

Aging and Balance

I think we all know that problems with falling—and worrying about falling—are common in older people. This is because aging affects all of your balance systems, as well as your ability to respond quickly and appropriately to balance challenges. But because so many factors contribute to your ability to balance, you can often compensate for losses in one area by cultivating other aspects of balance. So let's take a closer look at how aging affects each of those factors and which ones you can influence with your yoga practice.

VESTIBULAR SYSTEM. The functioning of our inner ears gradually declines with age. The inner ear hair cells are unable to repair themselves and gradually die off, which ultimately affects your vestibular system's ability to keep you balanced. Although you cannot change your vestibular system itself, you can compensate for these losses by working on other aspects of balance, including your somatosensory system and your four essential physical skills.

VISION SYSTEM. Age-related changes to the lenses of your eyes make it harder to focus quickly. In addition, eye problems that become more common as we age, such as cataracts, loss of peripheral vision, glaucoma, and macular degeneration, negatively affect vision. Of course, for eye conditions that are helped by prescription glasses, wearing the glasses when you need to balance can help compensate for these losses. For conditions that glasses cannot help, you can compensate for loss of vision by using your vestibular and somatosensory systems to balance (after all, blind people can balance).

OTHER SENSES. Aging can gradually slow the relay of information between your brain and body, and this can affect both your sense of touch (your ability to take in information about the surface you're balancing on) and your proprioception (your awareness of where you are in a space).

A special problem often associated with aging is a lack of sensitivity in your feet. If you have spent years wearing shoes almost all the time, your feet become much less sensitive, which makes you less aware of the surface on which you're walking or balancing. But practicing yoga allows you to spend much more time with bare feet, and the poses where you stand on your bare feet, including all standing poses and balancing poses where you balance on one leg, will make your feet more sensitive and responsive.

A sedentary lifestyle or lack of variety in movement can reduce your proprioception over time, causing you to lose balance when you make an unusual movement. Yoga is very effective for improving proprioception because you practice a wide variety of poses and movements while focusing on your internal sensations.

STRENGTH. As we discussed in chapter 3, age-related muscle atrophy causes loss of strength over time. This loss of strength affects your ability to balance because if you get knocked off balance, you can't easily move back into balance. Improving your strength through a well-rounded yoga practice will also improve your ability to balance.

FLEXIBILITY. As we discussed in chapter 4, your muscles and joints become stiffer with age, so your range of motion is reduced. This stiffness can affect your ability to balance because you can't easily move from one position to another. So you can be knocked off balance more easily and will have a harder time moving back into balance afterward. Improving your flexibility through a well-rounded yoga practice will also help your ability to balance.

NERVOUS SYSTEM. Age-related changes to your nerves can cause them to relay information more slowly between your brain and body. This slowing of reaction time can affect your coordination and speed of movement, as well as the strength of your muscle responses, all of which will affect your balance. You can counteract the slowing of reaction time by frequently practicing balance poses—the repetition alone will help! You can also work on agility practices, initially starting at a slower pace and gradually increasing your speed over time.

In addition, the postural responses that keep you upright (or try to!) are a result of information sent to your brain from your eyes and inner ears, the pressure sensors on your feet, and your proprioceptors. So as we age, our postural reflexes can gradually slow down. Practicing a variety of yoga poses, especially poses that cultivate flexibility, balance, and agility, can improve postural reflexes that have become rusty from disuse and improve the speed of your responses.

How Yoga Helps

Fortunately, balance is a skill that you can cultivate, and the modern asana practice is one of the best disciplines we know for improving it. In addition to working on strength and flexibility—both of which are necessary for good balance—you can practice balancing itself in a wide variety of poses. And practicing in the safety of your yoga space allows you to challenge your balance in a controlled environment before you take on real-world challenges.

If your balance is currently shaky, you can use our variations of balance poses with props, such as chairs and walls, to improve your ability to balance comfortably and safely.

And for the times you do fall—hey, it happens to the best of us—your practice will increase your chances of falling "well." Baxter's yoga students who have fallen and lived to tell the tale report that their reaction times seemed faster, and they had the ability to choose how and where to fall. And often when they began to fall, they "caught themselves" before actually going all the way down.

Balance Poses

Balancing is a skill you can learn and relearn. Just practicing balance poses helps improve your balance. These poses will also improve your proprioception and sense of touch, your postural reflexes and reaction times, and your focus and confidence.

Because balance poses are an integral part of any active practice, you'll find that almost every active yoga practice includes one or more balance poses. Yoga balance poses include poses where you balance on other parts of your body besides one or two feet, including poses where you balance on two hands, on one hand and one foot (Side Plank Pose), on your shins (Hunting Dog Pose), on your sitting bones (Boat Pose), and so on.

There are many different ways of practicing the balance poses—some of which are accessible to people with poor balance—so you can gradually work your way from the easier versions to the more challenging ones. From there, you can add even more challenges, such as practicing with your eyes closed, varying the surface you're balancing on, and even making up your own poses.

Standing Poses

In addition to practicing balance poses, you can improve balance by practicing a wide variety of standing poses, which place your feet and your body in very different positions. For example, Warrior 1 Pose and Triangle Pose, with the front foot turned out and the back foot turned in and your pelvis in different positions over your legs, challenge your balance in surprising ways. Like balance poses, all these poses will improve your proprioception and sense of touch, your postural reflexes and reaction times, and your focus and confidence.

Sense of Touch and Proprioception

By practicing your yoga poses with bare feet, you improve the sense of touch on the bottom of your feet, which will aid your ability to balance in standing positions. (Spending more time with your shoes off in general will also help with this.) Once you are comfortable with your balance on a wood floor or a thin yoga mat, you can vary the surface on which you practice to further improve your sensitivity. You can also practice poses where you balance on other parts of your body to improve your sense of touch. Practicing mindfully—especially with an awareness of touch—will make you more sensitive overall, which is especially helpful when you're walking on slippery or uneven surfaces.

Doing a variety of poses takes your body into many different configurations, as does moving through flow sequences. Practicing without a mirror—which is typically how we do yoga—allows you to feel all those different positions from the inside out as you sense your own alignment without using your eyes. That will refine your proprioception. To take your proprioception to another level, you can work with subtle alignment cues or practice with your eyes closed. (To double-check your internal perception of your body position, you can use a mirror periodically or ask for feedback from your yoga teacher.)

Nervous System

You can use your asana practice to support the health of your somatic nervous system in general (see chapter 8) by practicing a wide variety of poses and movement patterns to activate all the nerves on a regular basis and by practicing balance and flow poses to keep your proprioceptors healthy. A regular active asana practice improves blood flow to your sensory nerve receptors and increases space around your nerves.

Confidence and Mental Focus

For some people, just plain fear of losing balance or even falling can compromise their ability or willingness to balance. But yoga allows you to challenge yourself in a safe, controlled environment. The ability to practice balance poses over and over—and when no one is looking—will help improve your confidence. If fear is a big problem, you can use stress management techniques (see chapter 9) to quiet your nervous system before working on your balance.

Practicing balance poses and moving through flow sequences trains your mind as you focus again and again on balancing. But you can also work specifically on mental focus by practicing meditation and breath practices (see chapter 10), which will benefit your balance both inside and outside the yoga room. To take it up a notch, you can even add "distraction" to your balance practice by practicing in a distracting environment, such as at the beach or with kids in the room, or by doing another task while you are balancing, such as tossing a ball from one hand to another.

USING YOGA FOR BALANCE

For those of you who are new to yoga—and to balance poses—our list of techniques includes a few basics to get you started. To safely explore balancing poses you have never done before, start by practicing the versions that use props or a wall for support before moving on to the classic pose. If you're fearful, you can practice any pose with your back near a wall so you can lean back against it if you feel yourself losing balance.

Those of you who have already mastered the basic balancing poses need to keep challenging yourselves if you want to keep improving your balance. So our list of techniques includes recommendations that will allow you to improve your balance for years to come.

Whatever your current level, you should practice poses that challenge your balance with a nonjudgmental attitude, as negative self-talk can sabotage you. As you start to practice, notice your thoughts. If they tend to be negative, such as "I suck at Tree Pose," try consciously taking a more neutral approach, such as, "Let's see what I can do today." Keep in mind that even if you do lose your balance, just by practicing your balance poses you are still benefitting tremendously, so practicing, rather than staying upright, is your real aim.

Techniques for Improving and Maintaining Balance

HOW OFTEN TO PRACTICE. Since you typically only practice a few balance poses in an active practice, it's a good idea to include one or more balance poses in every active practice that you do. However, to avoid injuries from overuse, make sure you vary which balance poses you practice. For example, if you're working on Tree Pose, do that only every other time and try a version of Warrior 3 Pose on alternate days.

HOW LONG TO HOLD THE POSES. Hold your balance poses until you notice your leg or whichever body part is supporting you is quivering and then try to hold for two to three seconds longer. Rest a few seconds before repeating on the other side. If you are only able to hold the pose for ten to thirty seconds, rest briefly after completing both sides and repeat the pose a second time. Over time, gradually work your way up to holds of one to two minutes.

BALANCE YOUR PRACTICE. To improve balance, it's important to practice a wide variety of balance poses as well as strength, flexibility, and agility poses throughout the week and month rather than just doing the same poses every day. Besides the standing balance poses, we recommend practicing yoga poses where you balance on other parts of your body. Try Side Plank Pose variations to work on your hands and the sides of your feet. Try Boat Pose variations to work on your sitting bones. Try Hunting Dog Pose to work on your shins as well as your hands. To keep your mind fully engaged and avoid relying on your body memory of past practices, vary the order in which you do your poses.

MINDFULNESS. Because maintaining awareness while you balance—rather than just throwing yourself into a balance pose and hoping for the best—is what will help you improve, you should mainly practice poses that are accessible enough so you can practice them mindfully. As you practice, focus on the sensations of being on and off balance and making whatever subtle adjustments are necessary to steady yourself. As you make progress with the accessible poses, you can gradually add in a few more challenging poses or variations.

To develop your proprioception, take time to really feel your own alignment in every single pose that you do. Are your arms even in Warrior 2 Pose? Are your knees actually straight in your standing poses? Is your head really aligned directly over your torso? Then take your proprioception to another level by working with more subtle alignment cues. For example, you could work with your shoulder blades, your collarbones, your inner thighs, or even something more esoteric, such as your psoas muscles (which run from your spine to your inner thighs). Sometimes there is an area you are not used to even sensing, and at first it will be hard to feel something there. But the more you bring your mind to the area, the easier it will be to sense it and eventually to move it.

CHALLENGING YOURSELF. It's important to continue to challenge your balance and keep moving to the edge of stability where you almost—or even do—lose your balance. You can do this by varying the poses you do, the way you use your vision, the type of surface you balance on, and the amount of distraction in your environment.

VARYING POSES. After mastering basic static poses and dynamic sequences, add more challenging poses and practices. You can search out new poses or variations, make up new versions of existing balance poses, or even invent your own balance poses. In general, you should progress from simple poses to more complex poses. After you master all the traditional poses, progress to inventing new versions that challenge your balance. For example, you could modify Tree Pose by shifting your hip toward your standing leg and tipping your torso and arms to your lifted leg side. To challenge yourself with balance in motion, progress to dynamic balance poses, such as dynamic Warrior 3 Pose, or create a dynamic sequence that combines two familiar balance poses, such as Tree Pose and Warrior 3 Pose.

REMOVING OR CHANGING VISION. After you're comfortable in a balance pose with your eyes open, you can take vision out of the equation. This helps improve both proprioception and your sense of touch as you have to rely on your internal sense of where you are in space as well as your vestibular system to balance. Try practicing in a darkened room, wearing sunglasses, or keeping your eyes completely closed. You can also change your vision by keeping your eyes open but changing the position of your head, by looking up or looking down, and by turning your head.

VARY THE SURFACE YOU BALANCE ON. Once you are comfortable balancing on a stable surface, such as a wood floor or a thin yoga mat, gradually move on to more and more unstable surfaces. Some possibilities include a rug or carpet, a foam mat, a foam block, and even a firm mattress. If it's possible to practice yoga outside, try some poses on the grass or sand. We also recommend practicing on an uneven surface, such as having half your foot on your mat and the other half directly on the floor.

CHANGING YOUR ENVIRONMENT. When you're ready for real-world challenges, you can try practicing in a distracting environment, such as at a park or the beach. You can also create a distracting environment in your yoga room by practicing with a talkative yoga friend or inviting some children or pets in to "help" you practice. You can also add "cognitive distraction drills" to your practice by chanting or even tossing a small ball or bean bag around while you balance.

EASY BALANCE PRACTICE

This sequence is designed as a starting practice for those who are new to yoga practice or who have poor balance. To gradually challenge and improve your balance, the poses progress from standing evenly on two feet, to standing asymmetrically, to standing on one foot and then move on to poses that involve balancing on other parts of your body, including your shin, hand, and sitting bones.

As you practice, maintain an even, steady breath and focus on bringing awareness to the parts of your body that touch the floor, keeping them stable.

If you worry about falling, practice near a wall so you can lean against it if you feel you are starting to fall. If you are feeling secure and want to challenge your balance more, try moving your gaze in Warrior 2 Pose and Triangle Pose.

For photos that illustrate the individual movements in Dynamic Arms Overhead Pose and Dynamic Warrior 2 Pose, see the "Dynamic Poses and Flow Sequences" section on page 282. For information on Equal Breath, see page 180.

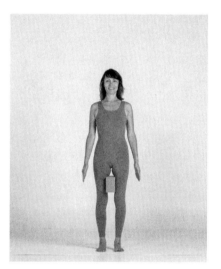

1. Mountain Pose, version 2, 30–90 seconds

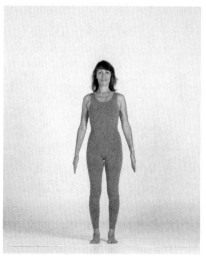

2. Mountain Pose, version 1, 30–90 seconds

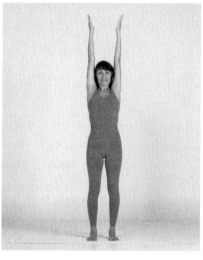

3. Dynamic Arms Overhead Pose, 6 times

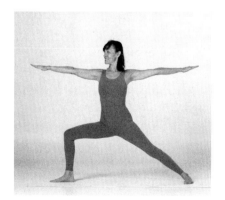

4. Warrior 2 Pose, any version, 30–90 seconds each side

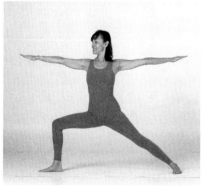

5. Dynamic Warrior 2 Pose, 6 times on each side

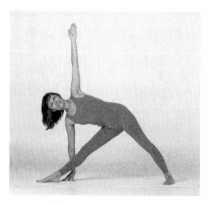

6. Triangle Pose, any version, 30–90 seconds each side

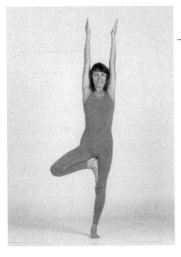

7. *Tree Pose, any version, 30–90 seconds each side*

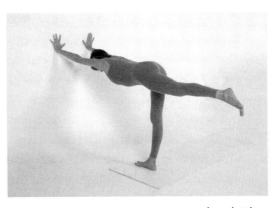

8. *Warrior 3 Pose, version 2, 30–90 seconds each side*

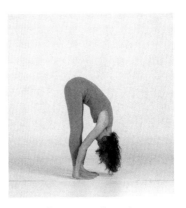

9. *Standing Forward Bend, any version, 30–60 seconds*

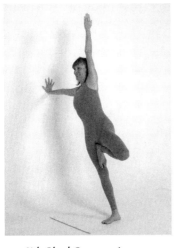

10. *Side Plank Pose, version 4, 30–60 seconds each side*

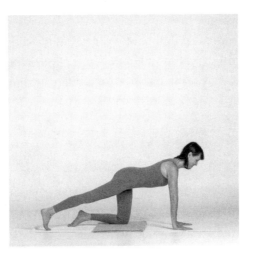

11. *Hunting Dog Pose, version 2, 30–90 seconds*

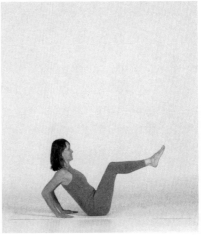

12. *Boat Pose, version 2, 30–90 seconds*

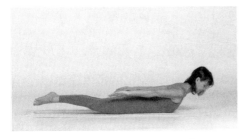

13. *Locust Pose, any version, 30 seconds, 2 times*

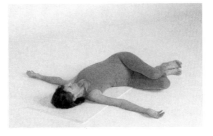

14. *Reclined Twist, version 1, 1–2 minutes each side*

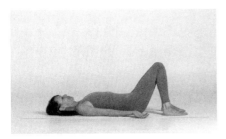

15. *Relaxation Pose, version 4, 1–2 minutes, equal breath practice for 12 breaths*

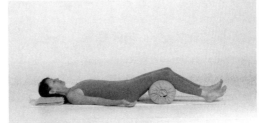

16. *Relaxation Pose, version 3, 5–10 minutes*

CHALLENGING BALANCE PRACTICE

This sequence assumes that you can do the Easy Balance Practice with some ease and focuses on more advanced balance poses and flow sequences that will help you take your balance abilities to a new level. To add extra challenge, we recommend that you practice some of the standing poses, such as Arms Overhead Pose and Extended Side Angle Pose, with your eyes closed. As those get easier, try closing your eyes in the other static poses, such as Warrior 1 Pose, Boat Pose, and Side Plank Pose. As you maintain each pose, focus your attention on creating a sense of stability and ease. The sequence winds down with Child's Pose and a session of alternate nostril breathing to balance your energy after a challenging practice.

You can find photos for Extended Side Angle Vinyasa in the "Dynamic Poses and Flow Sequences" section on page 282 and instructions for practicing alternate nostril breathing on page 181.

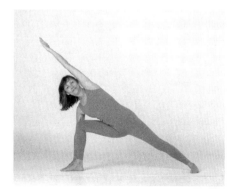

1. Arms Overhead Pose, version 2, 30–90 seconds

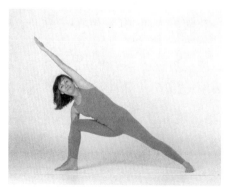

2. Arms Overhead Pose, version 2, 30–90 seconds, with eyes closed

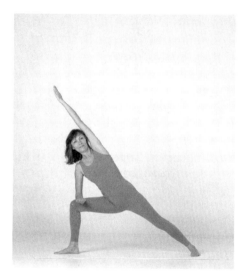

3. Extended Side Angle Pose, version 2, 30–90 seconds each side

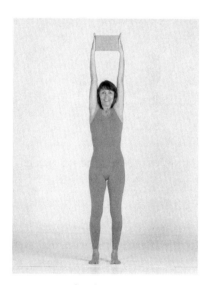

4. Extended Side Angle Vinyasa, 3 times each side

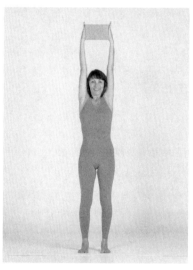

5. Extended Side Angle Pose, any version, 30–60 seconds each side, with eyes closed

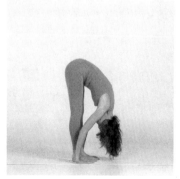

6. Standing Forward Bend, any version, 30–90 seconds

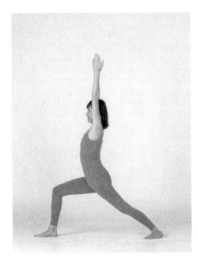

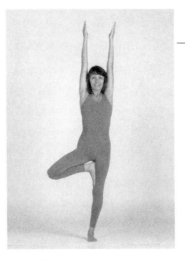

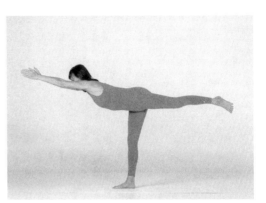

7. Warrior 1 Pose, version 1, 2 or 3, 30–60 seconds each side

8. Tree Pose, version 1, 3, or 4, 30–90 seconds each side

9. Warrior 3 Pose, version 1, 3, or 4, 30–90 seconds each side

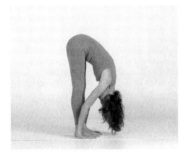

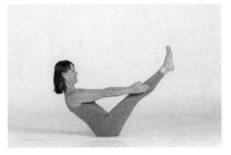

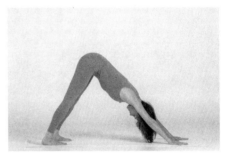

10. Standing Forward Bend, any version, 30 seconds

11. Boat Pose, version 1, 3, or 4, 30–90 seconds, 2 times

12. Downward-Facing Dog Pose, any version, 1 minute

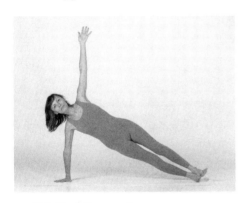

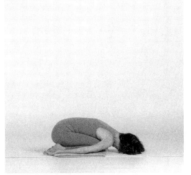

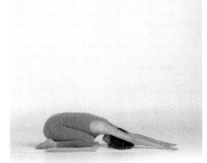

13. Side Plank Pose, version 1, 2 or 3, 30–60 seconds each side

14. Child's Pose, version 1 or 2, 1 minute

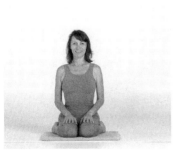

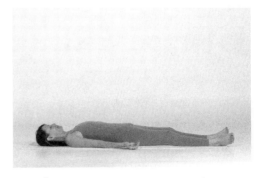

15. Hero Pose, any version, 2–4 minutes, alternate nostril breath, 2 sets of 6 cycles

16. Relaxation Pose, any version, 5–10 minutes

6

Yoga for Agility

AGILITY IS THE ABILITY TO MOVE EASILY THROUGH A SERIES OF positions while you stay balanced and in control. It's our fourth essential physical skill because it is necessary for many everyday situations, such as getting in and out of a car (especially the back seat of a two-door model!) and getting down to and up from the floor. Besides these basic movements, chances are you'll want to be able to continue doing more tricky maneuvers, such as getting in and out of a kayak, walking down a steep, rocky path, or squeezing yourself and your suitcase into a crowded train. Often speed, as well as coordination, is required, as when you walk down a crowded city sidewalk or scoop up a ball that's rolling along the ground. For those of you who dance, practice movement arts, or play sports, maintaining agility can improve your overall skills. Maintaining agility also helps prevent falls, which can be a serious problem for older people.

At age sixty-seven, Nina Rook credits her yoga-given agility for providing her with the confidence to spend time out in nature. Because in addition to gazing at the Persiads, being mobbed by chipmunks, and watching river otters, ravens, and pikas, for her being out in nature means loading cars, putting up and breaking down tents, finding firewood, and hauling water.

Before taking up yoga, she was strong, with good stamina and endurance, but her shaky balance, inflexibility, and inattentiveness led to more than her share of sprains, strains, and injuries from torqued knees. She says that it was only when she started a regular yoga practice that she realized other things were within her reach, both figuratively and literally: "the furthest plum on the branch I was trying to harvest."

Ultimately her yoga-given agility allowed her to singlehandedly dock a boat against a fast-moving current, a task that requires judging distances and speeds, stilling the boat as much as possible, jumping out at the right second with cleat in one hand and line in the other, and quickly securing the boat to the dock. All of this, Nina Rook says, is "about as far from my original, rigid, unbalanced roots as I could hope to be."[1]

ABOUT AGILITY

Being agile and coordinated requires a combination of physical and mental skills. To start, you need all three of the other essential skills that you're already working on: strength, flexibility, and balance. Your ability to make coordinated, precise movements also depends on how you interact with your external environment. As we discussed in chapter 5, your somatosensory system, which includes your basic five senses (vision, hearing, touch, taste, and smell) and proprioception (your ability to tell where one body part is in relation to another), allows you to maintain your balance in a static position as well as sense where your body is in space as you move from one position to another. So all are as important for agility as they are for balance.

Touch and Proprioception

When you're holding a pose, your sense of touch helps you keep your balance; when you're moving, it helps you take in information about the surface you're moving across—a sandy beach, a cobblestone street, or a rocky path in the mountains—so your brain knows what types of actions to take to help you stay balanced.

And the same sense of proprioception you use to maintain balance is needed for maintaining agility. Knowing where your body is in space, which direction you are heading, how fast you are going, and where the parts of your body are in relation to each other are essential for moving from one position to another with speed and grace. For example, when you're stepping out of the car with one foot in front of you and one foot behind you, you don't want to have to look around to see what your back leg is doing! Or, if you're doing a Sun Salutation and stepping from Standing Forward Bend into a Lunge Pose, you need to be able to move your back leg by sensing where it is in space.

Vision and Hearing

When you are moving, you need your eyes and ears as well as your proprioception to tell you where you are in space. For example, when you're getting out of a car, you use your eyes to tell you where to move your legs to get them through the door. You also need your eyes and ears to provide you with information about possible obstacles and your relationship to them. Imagine walking down a crowded sidewalk during your lunch hour, hiking a mountain path, or doing Sun Salutations in a crowded classroom: Is that someone riding a skateboard behind you? Is that rock in the middle of the path over there slippery? Should you step back a bit so you don't hit that person next to you when you bring your arms out to the sides?

Focus

Unless you're doing a series of movements that have become automatic, your ability to concentrate as you move from one position to another is a very important aspect of agility. Becoming distracted can throw you off balance or cause you to run into an obstacle. Let's say you're at a music festival weaving your way through the obstacle course of other people, their blankets, chairs, and coolers, and toddlers bolting off in random directions. Just imagine what would happen if you stopped looking where you were going or paying attention to where you were placing your feet!

Even for a routine set of movements, such as in a Sun Salutation, some amount of mental focus is needed, as complete distraction causes you to lose track of where you are or suddenly find yourself doing the wrong thing.

Speed

For those times when you need to respond quickly as well as with coordination, your strength is particularly important. Because the fast-twitch fibers in your muscles affect the speed and explosiveness of your muscle contractions, strong muscles provide you with both power and velocity. Moving with speed on a regular basis will prepare you for those situations when being agile means responding quickly. A healthy somatic nervous system is also important for speed. This is the part of your nervous system that allows voluntary control of your body movements and quick, coordinated responses to your mental requests for movement (see chapter 8 for more information).

Before discussing how you can use yoga to improve your agility, let's have a look at how aging affects this essential physical skill.

Agility and Aging

Because agility requires balance in motion, all of the age-related changes that affect balance affect your agility as well. And because rapid, coordinated movement requires strength and flexibility, age-related changes that reduce either strength or flexibility will also have a negative effect on agility. So using your asana practice to work on balance, strength, and flexibility, as well targeting agility specifically, will help you maintain your overall agility as you age.

Speed and Strength. Although age-related muscle atrophy negatively impacts both slow-twitch muscle fibers (which affect endurance) and fast-twitch muscle fibers (which affect the speed and explosiveness of your muscle contractions), we tend to lose more fast-twitch fibers as we age. So using your yoga practice to maintain strength is an especially important way of maintaining the speed you need for agility.

Nervous System. The aging of your nervous system gradually reduces the speed at which the nerves relay information between your brain and body. This means that it takes longer for your body to take action after you make the decision to move. Naturally this has an impact on your ability to move with coordination and speed. So using your yoga practice to maintain the health of your nervous system (see chapter 8) is especially important for maintaining agility.

How Yoga Helps

A well-rounded yoga practice that cultivates strength, flexibility, and balance provides the basic foundation for enhancing your agility. Just learning a wide range of yoga poses helps you maintain and even increase agility because the subtle movements you make stimulate your proprioceptors, the nerve endings in your joints and muscles that tell your brain where you are in space, which direction you are heading, and how fast you are going. This increased body awareness will aid you not only in mastering your yoga poses but also in every other physical activity. Yoga also enables you to work directly on your agility by focusing on coordination and speed.

Dynamic Poses and Flow Sequences

Moving dynamically in and out of a pose with your breath or between linked poses in flow sequences allows you to practice quick, precise movements.

This improves your overall coordination and exercises the fast-twitch fibers that assist in quick movements. The wide range of dynamic poses and flow sequences available (and the ability to make up new ones!) provides you with enough variability to address nearly all of your muscles and to stay challenged. By learning new sequences of yoga postures—especially dynamic sequences, when you change poses after just a few breaths—you challenge and improve your coordination and response time. Even making small changes in flow sequences will encourage you to stay attentive and nimble.

Static Poses

Moving in and out of static poses with precision helps improve coordination, and making subtle adjustments to your alignment while you're in a pose refines your ability to sense where you are in space and improves fine motor control (as you start to use rarely used muscles). The large variety of static poses plus their many variations means you can use virtually all of your muscles—in many different ways—throughout a given week rather than just doing the same basic movements over and over.

FLOOR POSES. Getting down to and up from the floor on a regular basis helps you maintain agility (and it's one of the things you need agility for!). So adding floor poses to your practice is beneficial, even if you have to use support to get up and down.

Mindfulness and Focusing

For all poses, practicing mindfully engages and refines your senses. You can observe the alignment of your body, listen to the sounds your body makes as you move and breathe, and notice how your body feels interacting with the environment—the floor, the walls, the air in the room—and how it feels when one body part touches another. Practicing mindfully also improves your proprioception, as you observe your alignment and learn to make subtle adjustments to it.

MENTAL FOCUS. Moving through flow sequences trains your mind as you return your focus again and again to making quick, precise movements while maintaining balance. In addition, meditation and breath practices (see chapter 10) can improve your mental focus in general, benefitting your agility both inside and outside the yoga room.

COGNITIVE DISTRACTION. When you're ready for a real-world challenge, you can either add distractions to your home practice or take your agility practices into a distracting environment, such as a public park or beach. Nina has been known to do Sun Salutations at the airport!

USING YOGA FOR AGILITY

To improve agility, it's important to continue working on strength, flexibility, and balance. You can then build on that foundation by adding in agility practices, including flow sequences, such as Sun Salutations, and dynamic poses, such as the dynamic versions of Warrior 1 Pose, Warrior 2 Pose, and Warrior 3 Pose.

Techniques for Improving and Maintaining Agility

HOW OFTEN TO PRACTICE. We don't recommend practicing the same flow sequences every day (this could lead to overuse injuries), but if you are mixing your dynamic practices with static poses, it's a good idea to include one or two agility practices in every active practice you do. For safety's sake, just make sure that you don't do *the same* dynamic poses or flow sequences in every practice. So rather than doing Sun Salutations every day, include dynamic poses in your practice on alternate days.

BALANCE YOUR PRACTICE. To optimize your agility, practice as wide a variety of poses and sequences as possible. After you've practiced for a few years, you can even invent some new variations to keep things fresh and challenging. For example, you could link different poses together in your own flow sequences.

If you love doing Sun Salutations, try varying the flow a bit. For example, instead of stepping your foot straight back from Standing Forward Bend, step it to the outside edge of your mat and then step your second foot back to the opposite side of the mat, so you have a wider stance in Downward-Facing Dog Pose. Making these little changes can help keep your practice fresh and stimulating and also prepare you for the unpredictability of real-word challenges.

DYNAMIC POSES. When practicing dynamic poses, be clear about what your starting and full-pose positions are. Then choose an appropriate focus for the particular pose or practice. For instance, for Dynamic Warrior 2 Pose, you could bring attention to the bend of your front leg, aiming it straight ahead and stopping at 90 degrees. For Dynamic Bridge Pose, you could focus on keeping your breathing smooth as you move with precision between the two positions, coordinating the movements of your hips and arms with your breath.

HOW FAST TO MOVE. Varying your speed strengthens different muscle fibers. Faster movements use fast-twitch muscle fibers, which assist in strengthening muscles for more explosive movements as well as improving agility, while slower movements use slow-twitch muscle fibers, which lead to more overall strength and endurance.

So when you're practicing dynamic poses or flow sequences, it's a good idea to vary your speed—some days working slowly through your entire agility practice and others working at a faster pace. You can also do this within a given session, doing a set of dynamic repetitions slowly first and then repeating it at a faster pace.

STATIC POSES. Although they are not as effective for developing agility as dynamic poses, you can use your static poses to cultivate agility by moving in and out of the pose with care and precision. While you are in the pose, practice mindfully to improve your proprioception (see below).

FLOOR POSES. Do them! Do them every day! Get down to and up from the floor to do seated and reclined poses, even if you need to use a chair or the wall to help you get up and down. Look for opportunities to do this in your everyday life, too.

MINDFULNESS. To refine your senses of sight, hearing, and touch, choose one sense to focus on in a given practice. Use your eyes to verify your alignment. Are your feet evenly aligned on the floor or is one foot really turned out? Use your ears to listen to your breath or note how gracefully or awkwardly you make certain movements—when you step into a new position, are you coming down lightly or heavily? Feel how evenly you are pressing into the floor or onto a prop and notice when one part of your body is touching another (sometimes this means you're doing the pose right and other times—oops!).

IMPROVE PROPRIOCEPTION. To improve agility, focus on improving your proprioception in all of your poses. In static poses, take some time to really feel your own alignment. Are your arms even in Warrior 2 Pose? Are your knees actually straight in your standing poses? Is your head really aligned directly over your torso? In dynamic poses, you can either focus on a single movement or on keeping your breathing smooth as you coordinate breath and movement.

To take your proprioception to another level, work with more subtle alignments, such as your shoulder blades, collarbones, inner thighs, or even psoas muscles. Sometimes there is an area you are not used to sensing but the more you bring your mind to it, the easier it will be to sense that area and eventually to move it.

Taking vision out of the equation helps improve proprioception because you'll need to *sense* where your body is in a space to compensate for lack of sight. That's how you walk in the dark! You can experiment by practicing in a darkened room or keeping your eyes closed.

COGNITIVE DISTRACTION. Although you can't toss a ball around while you do agility practices the way you can in balance poses, you can play music or talk radio, invite some pets or children into your yoga room, or practice out in a park or at the beach.

EASY AGILITY PRACTICE

This sequence is designed to improve your agility by combining dynamic poses that allow you to move in and out of poses with some speed (take them at your own pace) and static poses that allow you to develop precision in the way you slowly move into and out of the poses.

As you practice the sequence, focus on making smooth transitions while maintaining your balance and keeping your breath smooth and even. When you practice the mini Sun Salutations, the first time through step back into Lunge Pose with your right foot. Then, when you return from Downward-Facing Dog Pose to Lunge Pose, step forward with your right foot. The second time through, lead with your left foot instead. Then alternate your lead foot for each round.

For photos that illustrate the individual movements in the dynamic poses and vinyasas, see the "Dynamic Poses and Flow Sequences" section on page 282.

CAUTION: If you have trouble with balance, work near a wall while doing this sequence so you can use it for support if necessary.

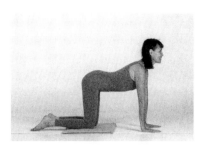

1. Dynamic Cat-Cow Pose, 6 times

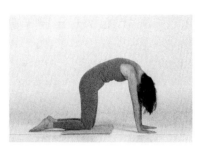

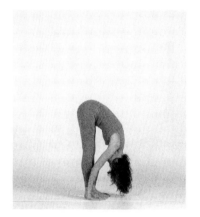

2. Hunting Dog Pose, version 1, 30–60 seconds each side

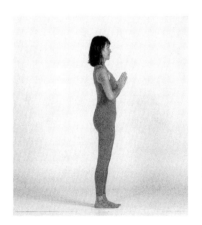

3. Dynamic Hunting Dog Pose, 6 times

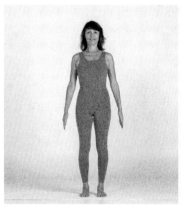

4. Mountain Pose, version 1, 1 minute

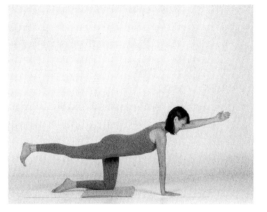

5. Standing Forward Bend Vinyasa, 6 times

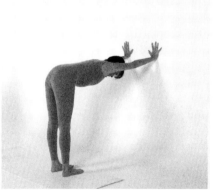

6. Mini Sun Salutations, 4 rounds

7. Half Downward-Facing Dog Pose, any version, 1 minute

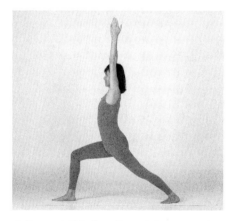

8. Dynamic Warrior 1 Pose, 6 times on each side

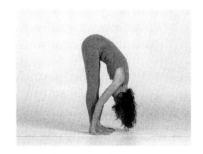

9. Standing Forward Bend, any version, 30–90 seconds

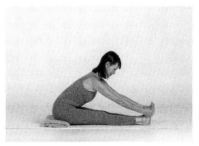

10. Seated Forward Bend, version 2, 1–3 minutes

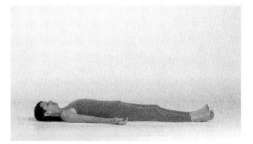

11. Relaxation Pose, any version, 5–10 minutes

CHALLENGING AGILITY PRACTICE

This sequence assumes that you can do the Easy Agility Practice with some ease and focuses on more advanced poses and flow sequences that will help you take your agility to a new level. Since agility is balance in motion, this practice contains several dynamic sequences, but it also includes a few static poses to return you to feeling stable and grounded. It ends with two restorative poses to allow you to rest and integrate your practice.

As you move through all the poses, focus on feeling balanced and maintaining a steady breath. When you practice the Sun Salutations, alternate sides by changing your lead foot, as in the Easy Agility Practice. For an added challenge, do them with your eyes closed or speed up your pace. After practicing Side Plank Pose, take a moment to shake out your hands and wrists before moving on to the next pose.

For photos that illustrate the individual movements in Dynamic Downward-Facing Dog, Extended Side Angle Vinyasa, Side Plank Vinyasa, Dynamic Reclined Twist, and Dynamic Bridge Pose, see "Dynamic Poses and Flow Sequences" section on page 282.

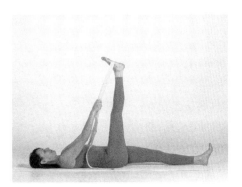

1. Reclined Leg Stretch, versions 1 and 3, 1 minute each side

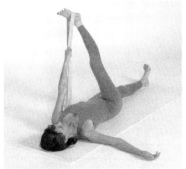

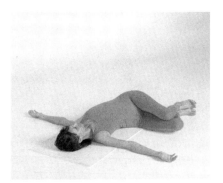

2. Dynamic Reclined Twist, 6 times

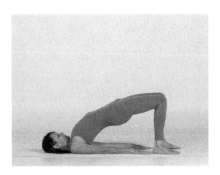

3. Dynamic Bridge Pose, 6 times

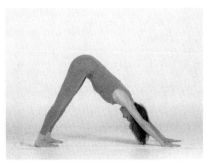

4. Dynamic Downward-Facing Dog Pose, 6 times

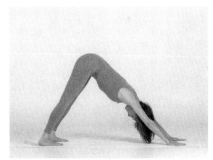

5. Downward-Facing Dog Pose, any version, 30 seconds

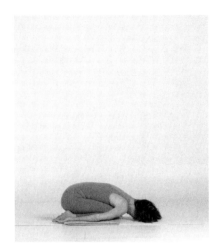

6. Childs's Pose, any version, 30–60 seconds

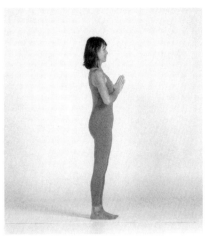

7. Mini Sun Salutations, 2 rounds

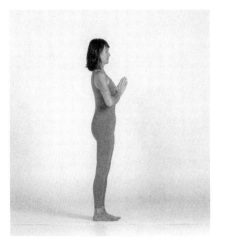

8. Full Sun Salutations, 2 rounds. Hold Upward-Facing Dog Pose for 2–3 breaths

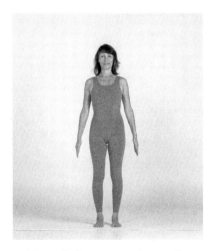

9. Mountain Pose, any version, 1 minute

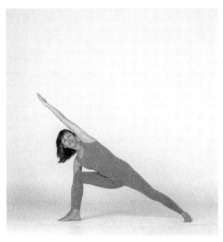

10. Extended Side Angle Vinyasa, 2 rounds, alternating sides

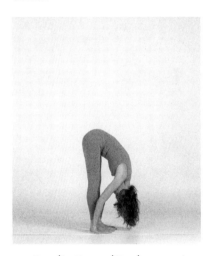

11. Standing Forward Bend, any version, 30 seconds

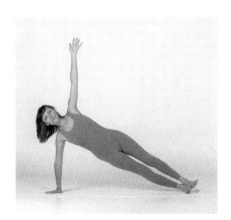

12. Side Plank Vinyasa, 6 times, alternating sides

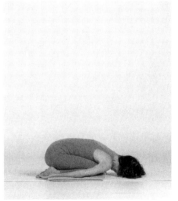

13. Child's Pose, any version, 1–2 minutes

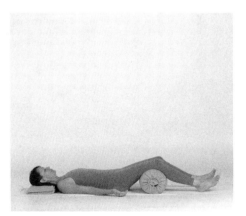

14. Relaxation Pose, version 3, 5–10 minutes

7

Heart and Cardiovascular System Health

Both sides of Victor Dubin's family have medically controlled high blood pressure. So it came as no surprise to him that at a medical checkup at age thirty-seven, he had blood pressure readings as high as 140/95. Because he had no other major risk factors, his doctor suggested that instead of taking medication he should monitor his blood pressure on a regular basis. This practice turned out to be an opportunity for mindfulness! In line with his newly found awareness, Victor consulted with a dietitian, modified his running routines, and made some simple yet dramatic changes to his yoga practice.

Most importantly, he started practicing yoga more regularly—five days per week, even if for just short periods of time. He noticed that the rare times when he skipped practice, he was more irritable, moody, and stressed, and his blood pressure reading was elevated, so he also began to emphasize inverted poses in his practice because they are particularly beneficial for stress management, blood pressure regulation, and circulation. Finally, he made meditation and breath practices a priority by "front-loading" a sitting practice before moving through yoga poses, and he found these seated practices just as important for reducing blood pressure as physical exercise. Now he says:

Today, at age forty-three, my blood pressure reading is 113/74. It is my hope that my personal example of change and self-determination will be of support and inspiration to those of you who are engaged in similar struggles. You can make change, big change, and it can be made without tremendous shifts in your life. Laugh. Meditate. Breathe. Do some yoga (any yoga). Get outside. Think about what you are eating before, during, and after you eat it. Make commitments. Be consistent. Be dedicated. Be mindfully aware.[1]

Other changes Victor made besides changing his yoga practice included dramatically reducing his sodium intake, running more regularly, and having monthly acupuncture treatments and massage.

ABOUT YOUR HEART AND CARDIOVASCULAR SYSTEM

Your heart is just one component of an essential system that keeps you alive by delivering oxygen and nutrients throughout your entire body and carrying waste products to the organs responsible for elimination. Understanding a bit about how your entire cardiovascular system works will help you realize how important it is to use your yoga practice to keep your cardiovascular system functioning optimally.

Heart

Your heart, the organ at the center of your cardiovascular system, uses muscular contractions to pump blood throughout your body, supplying it with oxygen and other nutrients, hormones, and white blood cells and removing carbon dioxide and other waste products. The heart's built-in electrical system sets the rhythm of the muscular contractions, adjusting the rhythm as needed to accommodate your changing activities by staying in constant communication with your brain.

Blood and Blood Vessels

Your blood contains red and white blood cells, proteins, glucose, minerals, hormones, and platelets that help form scabs. When it is pumped from your heart through your blood vessels, it delivers oxygen, nutrients, hormones, and white blood cells throughout your body. It also retrieves waste products, which it moves to your kidneys and liver for processing, and hormones from various organs that are sending messages to your brain or other parts of your body.

Your blood vessels are tubes through which your heart pumps your blood, and they are named according to their function and size.

Arteries and arterioles. These transport nutrient-rich blood from your heart to capillaries and to your lungs to release carbon dioxide and receive oxygen. These blood vessels help maintain steady blood pressure by relaxing and contracting their walls.

Capillaries. With walls only one-cell thick, these blood vessels pass oxygen, nutrients, hormones, water, and salts into your body and receive carbon dioxide, waste products, salts, and hormones from it.

Veins and Venules. These blood vessels return blood from the capillaries back to your heart, first through smaller venules and then through larger veins. Because veins are not as thick or elastic as arteries, they partly rely on the natural squeezing action of your muscles when you are physically active to return your blood back to your heart. So being physically active is necessary for your veins to work most effectively.

Chest Cavity

Your chest cavity consists of your rib cage bones (your ribs, breastbone, and spine) and the muscles between your ribs and around your rib cage, which help you breathe and move your chest in general. Your heart resides within your chest cavity between your two lungs. When your chest cavity is healthy, with strong bones and strong and flexible muscles, your heart and lungs have the room they need to function optimally. However, poor posture or other conditions that affect the shape or health of your chest cavity, such as scoliosis, can compress your heart, impacting its ability to function.

Related Systems

Now we'll briefly look at some of the organs and systems that the cardiovascular system interacts with, so you can understand how using your yoga practice to support those systems can help your cardiovascular system. But keep in mind that the cardiovascular system interacts with everything in your body! No cell in your body is more than a few millimeters from a capillary because blood supplies nutrition to and removes waste from all cells, distributes hormones throughout the body as chemical messengers, and delivers white blood cells for immune system and repair jobs.

BRAIN AND NERVOUS SYSTEM. Depending on your activity level, your brain and nervous system make moment-by-moment adjustments to your heart rate and the force of your heartbeat as well as to your blood pressure. See chapter 8 for information on how to support brain and nervous system health.

RESPIRATORY SYSTEM. Your cardiovascular system circulates blood through your lungs to absorb oxygen that you've inhaled and then transports the oxygen-rich blood to the rest of your body. When your blood returns to your heart (after being cleaned by your liver and kidneys), your lungs absorb the carbon dioxide from your blood so you can exhale it. Healthy lung function is such an integral part of your cardiovascular system that some anatomists refer to the two systems together as the "cardio-respiratory system."

DIGESTIVE SYSTEM. Your cardiovascular system circulates through your intestines to absorb digested food in the form of sugar, fat, and proteins into your capillaries. It then transports the digested food to other organs for processing. For example, the cardiovascular system delivers sugar from the digestive system to the liver, which then converts it into storage particles for future use.

LIVER. In addition to storing glycogen, your liver filters your blood to metabolize drugs, break down old red blood cells to make bile, and remove various toxins. Without a healthy liver, your blood will gradually become toxic, which can lead to serious illness.

URINARY SYSTEM. Before your blood returns to your heart, your kidneys filter it, clearing waste and extra salt molecules, such as potassium and sodium, and moving them into urine for removal from your body. As with the liver, you need fully functional kidneys to keep your blood healthy.

SPLEEN. This organ filters out old red blood cells, recycles their iron, and helps clear bacteria from the blood. (It also provides a reservoir of about a pint of blood for release if your blood levels suddenly drop, such as if a major artery is cut.)

In this chapter we'll provide you with information about how you can use yoga to maintain the health of your entire cardiovascular system. If you're having problems with brain health and/or nervous system health, you should also use your yoga practice to support their health as well (see chapter 8). If you're having digestive problems, you can use yoga to manage chronic stress and support healthy eating (see chapter 9).

Before we discuss how you can use yoga to maintain cardiovascular health, let's have a look at how aging affects this essential system, so you'll understand what you can influence with your yoga practice.

The Cardiovascular System and Aging

For most people, the age-related changes to the cardiovascular system described in this section occur gradually over time and typically result in minimal to moderate loss of function. So most people will not see a significant impact on their daily activities. Of course this is not true for everyone, and a smaller percentage of people—including, but not limited to, people with certain genetic tendencies—do develop more serious conditions. Because these age-related conditions are serious, it makes good sense for all of us to take preventative measures. By learning a bit about these age-related changes, you will better understand why yoga is so beneficial for fostering heart and cardiovascular health and know which practices to choose to gain the appropriate benefits.

HEART. As the heart ages, the cardiac muscle gradually stiffens and weakens. In a small percentage of people, if this weakness reaches a critical level, the muscle thickens, which can lead to congestive heart failure. Maintaining a regular exercise program, eating a healthy diet, and avoiding smoking may all help lower your chances of developing this problem.

The heart's electrical system gradually begins to work less efficiently. For some people this can cause heartbeats to slow down, speed up, or beat irregularly. Heartbeats that are too fast, too slow, or irregular may cause weakness, dizziness, palpitations, or, in extreme cases, fainting, all of which could reduce the ability to exercise or even go about daily activities. Exercising, managing stress, maintaining a healthy diet, and regularly resting your heart may prevent these problems from developing in the first place. For those with symptoms, these lifestyle changes may improve the functioning of the heart's electrical system.

BLOOD. Because aging reduces the fluid in your bloodstream, your overall blood volume gradually decreases, and the number of red blood cells that you produce in response to stress or illness is also decreased, which can slow your response to blood loss or anemia. Although the production of most of your white blood cells remains the same, those that provide immunity decrease both in number and capacity, which can impact your ability to resist infection. Maintaining a healthy diet, keeping well hydrated, and staying physically active can help minimize these changes.

BLOOD VESSELS. The walls of the blood vessels that feed your heart and circulate throughout your entire body gradually stiffen. In some people these vessels also narrow because of plaque deposits, which makes it harder to deliver nourishment and remove waste. The combination of stiffening and narrowing of these blood vessels in some may eventually lead to heart attacks or heart pain (angina), high blood pressure, increased risk of strokes, and decreased exercise tolerance. Fortunately, exercising, managing stress, maintaining a healthy diet, and doing inverted poses that assist the return of blood to the heart can improve your circulation and help keep blood vessels healthy, which may prevent these serious conditions from developing. For those who already have clogged blood vessels around the heart, studies indicate that you can reverse these changes with the same combination of exercise, stress management, and healthy diet.

How Yoga Helps

Because yoga includes active exercise, resting poses, and stress management practices, it's particularly effective for maintaining heart and overall cardiovascular system health. You can use your practice to exercise and rest your heart and maintain the health of your chest cavity, and you can improve circulation, reduce chronic stress (which causes the heart and cardiovascular system to overwork and may contribute to the development of heart disease, high blood pressure, and stroke), and maintain the health of the organs and systems your cardiovascular system depends on. We'll address each of these benefits in detail next.

CAUTION: In this chapter we are providing recommendations for using yoga tools for their preventative benefits. Start by considering the health status of your heart and cardiovascular system. If you're healthy, then you can follow our recommended techniques, but if you're having cardiovascular problems or have risk factors for developing heart problems, such as untreated hypertension (high blood pressure), coronary artery disease, or angina, you should consult your doctor or your cardiologist about whether you can practice yoga. If your doctor clears you to try yoga, we recommend you then consult with a yoga therapist or a yoga teacher who is experienced with teaching people with your particular condition.

Exercising Your Heart

For exercising your heart, you can use a combination of active static poses and dynamic poses or flow sequences.

STATIC POSES. Poses that you hold for thirty seconds or more increase your heart's workload, which strengthens the heart muscle itself. (If you have high blood pressure, please approach these poses with caution and work into long holds very gradually, preferably under the guidance of an experienced teacher.)

DYNAMIC POSES AND FLOW SEQUENCES. If you practice slowly, moving in and out of poses with your breath gradually warms up your body and your cardiovascular system. If you practice more quickly, moving in and out of poses with your breath increases your heart rate, providing you with aerobic exercise.

In general, we recommend practicing a combination of both static poses with longer holds and dynamic poses and sequences that you can practice at a rapid pace after first warming up.

Resting Your Heart

Even if you're not experiencing chronic stress, it's as beneficial for you to rest your heart and cardiovascular system as it is to exercise it. Because restorative poses practiced with a mental focus and gentle inverted poses slow your heart rate and lower your blood pressure, they're ideal poses for resting both your heart muscle and its electrical system. During times of intensive physical activity, busyness, or stress, a restful yoga practice can provide a healthy break during your day. See chapter 9 for information on restorative yoga.

Improving Your Circulation

PUMPING ACTION. A well-rounded active yoga practice supports the efficient flow of blood throughout your cardiovascular system. When you move your body through a series of yoga poses, you are contracting and relaxing most of your muscles. This improves your circulation in general, as it helps your heart pump blood through your arteries and veins.

This pumping action is especially helpful for your veins because to return blood back to your heart, they partly rely on the natural contracting and relaxing of your muscles that happens only when you're active. The pumping action can also help move the blood in stagnant areas in varicose veins (weak veins that prevent the return of blood to the heart) back toward your heart.

For dynamic poses, repeatedly moving in and out of the pose with your breath does an excellent job on its own of creating the pumping action to improve your circulation. Sun Salutations and Dynamic Warrior 2 Pose would work well for this purpose.

For static poses, moving in and out of the pose once creates a pumping action that is obviously less effective than moving in and out of the pose repeatedly. However, when you are practicing static poses for their other benefits, you can enhance the pumping action by rhythmically contracting and relaxing as many muscle groups as possible while you're in the pose. For example, you could practice Triangle Pose or Warrior 2 Pose while consciously contracting and relaxing your leg and arm muscles.

INVERTED POSES. Poses where your legs are higher than your heart, such as Legs Up the Wall Pose or even Reclined Leg Stretch, are especially beneficial for improving circulation because in these positions gravity helps the veins move the blood down toward your heart. These poses can also help reduce swelling in your legs.

BLOOD VESSEL HEALTH. In general, the exercise you get from a well-rounded active practice that includes both static and dynamic poses will help maintain the health of the blood vessels themselves, as exercise and improved blood flow help keep the blood vessels from hardening.

Reducing Chronic Stress

Chronic stress has a serious impact on your heart and cardiovascular system health. Being in a constant state of low-level stress overworks your heart and cardiovascular system, which can lead to the development of heart disease and/or high blood pressure.

The yoga stress management practices we recommend in chapter 9 reduce chronic stress, which can help prevent heart disease and high blood pressure and keep your heart's electrical system healthy. If you already have high blood pressure, you can try using these techniques to lower your blood pressure, although you should check with your doctor first before trying them.

Stress management techniques also reduce inflammation, which is now thought to be a primary cause of clogged arteries. Because inflammation also contributes to the hardening of blood vessels, managing chronic stress will also maintain the health of your blood vessels overall.

Stress management can also help you maintain a healthy weight, which is important for heart health because obesity is a frequent cause of heart disease, high blood pressure, and other circulatory system problems. Because stress causes high levels of cortisol, which in turn causes stress eating and weight gain, reducing chronic stress will lower your cortisol levels, which can help with weight management.

All the stress management techniques are equally helpful for your heart and cardiovascular system's health, so you should focus on practicing the ones that suit your current health conditions and preferences. If stress is an ongoing problem for you, cultivating equanimity—which allows you to stay balanced during periods of difficulty—will keep you from becoming too stressed out in the first place. See chapter 10 for several different ways to cultivate equanimity. You can use any equanimity practice that works for you—and doesn't cause you to stress out when you try it.

Victor said that he found meditating on certain topics especially helpful for lowering his blood pressure:

> While many topics of meditation/contemplation had a positive effect on lowering my blood pressure, some that seemed to lower it most and most consistently are thinking of my loved ones and how I love them, broadening my view of nature and the natural world, and whatever makes me smile.[2]

Healthy Eating

We think you all know by now that a healthy diet is important for heart and cardiovascular health. Although it's beyond the scope of this book to go into the topic in detail, we have some suggestions on using yoga for healthy eating in chapter 9.

USING YOGA FOR HEART AND CARDIOVASCULAR SYSTEM HEALTH

This section provides recommendations for using your yoga practice as a preventative tool for fostering heart and cardiovascular health. If you are already practicing well-rounded active sequences that include a few restorative poses (or at the least a long Relaxation Pose), breath work, and meditation, that's a great start because regular exercise and stress management both help support heart and cardiovascular health. The following sections provide additional recommendations for those who want to focus especially on these areas.

Techniques for Improving and Maintaining Heart and Cardiovascular System Health

HOW OFTEN TO PRACTICE. In general, we recommend that you practice five to six days a week to promote cardiovascular health. Practice a vigorous sequence, including active poses and/or flow sequences, at least three days a week but no more than every other day (your body needs time for recovery and repair). On other days, practice gentle or restorative sequences, which are safe to practice every day, or pranayama, meditation, or philosophy studies, which are also safe on a daily basis.

HOW LONG TO PRACTICE. If you are newer to yoga, start out with shorter sessions of ten to fifteen minutes. Then, if your schedule allows, gradually lengthen the amount of time you spend each day in practice, working your way up to thirty- to sixty-minute sessions to increase the effects of both exercising and resting your cardiovascular system. If you are a more experienced practitioner, you can start off with longer practices of thirty to sixty minutes. Feel free to shorten or lengthen a practice on any given day to accommodate changes in your work and home schedules.

BALANCE YOUR PRACTICE. To vary the effects on your heart and circulatory system, we recommend that you include both static poses and dynamic poses and sequences in your practices. Also include gentle and restorative poses to rest your heart and lower overall stress. Try to allocate a few minutes, either at the beginning or end of your practice, for simple breath work, including stimulating practices to work your heart and calming practices to rest your heart (see chapter 10 for information on both these types of practices). Finally, remember to practice Relaxation Pose, either with simple breath awareness or with a guided relaxation recording, to finish your practice.

It's also a good idea to include a short meditation of three to five minutes at the start or end of your practice, or both. (Of course, you can always meditate at another time in the day, if that works better for you.)

STRESS MANAGEMENT. One of the most effective ways to influence your cardiovascular system over time is to practice stress management techniques, such as meditation or restorative yoga, every day or as often as you can manage (see chapter 9 for a complete selection of techniques). None of these techniques is inherently more effective than any other, but you may find that one or two work best for you. We recommend that you try them all at some point, so you can choose the right one for you for a particular day or period of time in your life. You can practice any of these stress management techniques as part of your regular asana practice or alone, at a different time of day.

STATIC POSES. The more physically challenging a pose is, the greater the workload on your heart, which is a particularly good way to exercise your heart and cardiovascular system. So try to practice the following on a regular basis:

- Standing poses that are challenging for you to maintain, such as the Warrior poses and Extended Side Angle Pose
- Poses where you bear weight on your arms, such as Plank Pose, Side Plank Pose, and Downward- and Upward-Facing Dog poses
- Any strength-building poses
- Inverted poses (see below)

HOW LONG TO HOLD POSES. If you are newer to yoga, start out with shorter holds of three to six breaths and gradually work up to longer holds of 90 to 120 seconds over time. If you are an experienced practitioner, hold the poses until you become slightly fatigued and gradually work your way up to longer holds.

DYNAMIC POSES AND FLOW SEQUENCES. If you are not already practicing dynamic poses or flow sequences, we recommend that you get used to continuous movement by starting with simple dynamic poses, such as Dynamic Arms Overhead Pose, Dynamic Easy Sitting Twist, or Dynamic Cat-Cow Pose for six to ten rounds. After that, you can move on to more challenging dynamic poses and our shorter flow sequences that combine two or more linked poses. When you're ready for the classic flow sequences, mini or full Sun Salutations, we recommend starting out with two to four rounds and gradually working up to ten to twenty rounds.

Start by doing these poses and sequences at a leisurely pace, with a comfortable breath rate. After you become accustomed to practicing dynamically, you can gradually pick up your pace to increase the work on your cardiovascular system, which will increase your heart and breath rates. Assess how your body is handling the new pace and slow down if necessary. If you are a more experienced practitioner, you can challenge yourself by starting out at a faster pace than you normally would. But you, too, should assess how your body is handling the new pace and make any necessary adjustments.

INVERTED POSES. Because inverted poses help return blood from the parts of your body that are below your heart and can have a positive effect on your blood pressure feedback system, we recommend that you include these poses in your practices. Be sure to include active inverted poses, even partial ones, such as Downward-Facing Dog Pose and Standing Forward Bend. Work your way gradually up to longer holds of 90 to 120 seconds, as you would with other active poses.

We also recommend that you practice supported inverted poses, such as Legs Up the Wall Pose and Supported Bridge Pose, two to three times per week. You can include these in your active practices, practice them as part of a restorative practice, or even practice them on their own. (See chapter 9 for information on supported inverted poses and how long to hold them.)

RESTORATIVE POSES. We recommend that you include one or two restorative poses in your active practices, at either the beginning or the end. We also recommend that you practice a full restorative sequence periodically to fully rest your heart and cardiovascular system. Try this once a week to start with. If you enjoy it, do it more often. (See chapter 9 for information on restorative yoga and how long to hold the poses.)

EQUANIMITY PRACTICES. Because equanimity practices may help you avoid getting stressed out in the first place, they are helpful for promoting heart and cardiovascular health. Read chapter 11 and then experiment to determine which equanimity practices work best for you. Then practice as often as you can, even daily if possible.

The Importance of Regular Practice

Remember Victor Dubin's dramatic story at the beginning of this chapter about how he lowered his high blood pressure? He reported that one of the most important changes he made in his routine was simply to start practicing yoga more regularly. Although he had been practicing for some time, before his blood pressure warning, his practice was "more haphazard and less consistent." After the warning, he took the advice he often gives to others that "80% of the benefit of doing yoga comes from just doing yoga." Because he believes in the common saying that "the perfect is the enemy of the good," he established a new routine of doing a little bit of yoga five days per week no matter what, designing his practice schedule to fit in with his family responsibilities. This is how he describes it:

> At that time I needed to start prepping breakfast and lunches at 7:30 a.m. So I decided that my practice would start at whatever time it could and always end at 7:30. Some mornings I would get up and start practicing by 6:30, but most mornings I would start around 7:05. Sometimes I wouldn't be able to start until 7:26 and I would contemplate just scrapping it altogether, but then I realized that the routine mattered more than the duration. So I would practice for three or four minutes and then end at 7:30.

Other times when I did end up scrapping the practice altogether for the day, I would be more irritable, moody, stressed, and inevitably my blood pressure readings would be elevated. In other words, even just three or four minutes made a dramatic impact in lowering my blood pressure! Don't get me wrong, I am not starting a new fad of "3 Minute Yoga!" There are times when a longer practice really helps and makes a bigger difference. I'm simply suggesting that an all or nothing attitude is ultimately destructive."[3]

So even though we've just recommended a lot of different techniques for fostering cardiovascular system and heart health and we're including a full-length sequence for you to practice below, we suggest keeping Victor's approach in mind. Regular practice—even if that means just a short session of Legs Up the Wall Pose—is more important than skipping practice on a day when you can't manage to find a free hour.

CARDIOVASCULAR HEALTH PRACTICE

This sequence is designed to help you maintain or improve your cardio-vascular health by combining challenging static poses that increase the workload of your heart and dynamic sequences to exercise your heart muscle aerobically. The sequence also includes supported inversions to improve circulation and reduce stress, and a Child's Pose to rest your heart. It concludes with a calming breath practice for additional stress management.

As you practice the poses, focus on maintaining a steady breath and a feeling of vitality in your heart area. In Legs Up the Wall Pose, visualize your heart as strong, steady, relaxed, and rested.

For the dynamic sequences, including mini Sun Salutations, Dynamic Warrior 2 Pose, and Dynamic Upward-Facing Dog Pose, move slowly at first and then gradually increase your pace. You can find the photos for these sequences in the "Dynamic Poses and Flow Sequences" section on page 282.

See page 176 for information on exhalation lengthening.

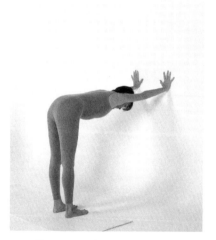

1. Half Downward-Facing Dog Pose, any version, 30–60 seconds, 2 times

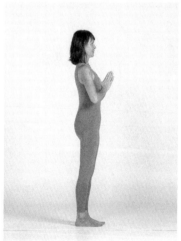

2. Mini Sun Salutations, 2–6 rounds

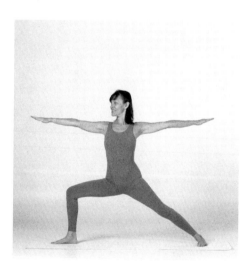

3. Dynamic Warrior 2 Pose, 6 times each side

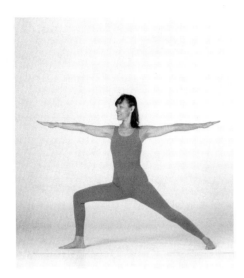

4. *Warrior 2 Pose, version 1, 2, or 3, 30–90 seconds each side*

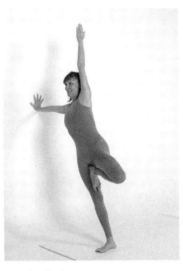

5. *Side Plank Pose, version 4, 30 seconds, 2 times each side*

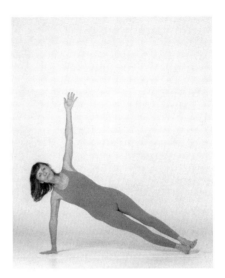

6. *Side Plank Pose, version 1, 30 seconds each side*

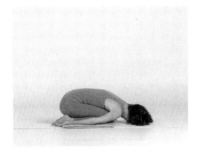

7. *Child's Pose, any version, 1 minute*

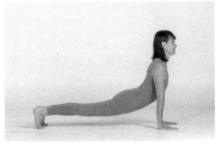

8. *Dynamic Upward-Facing Dog Pose, 3–6 times*

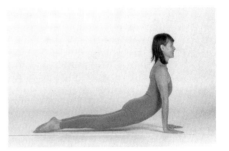

9. *Upward-Facing Dog Pose, any version, 10–30 seconds*

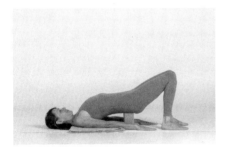

10. *Bridge Pose, version 2 or 3, 1–3 minutes*

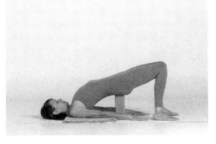

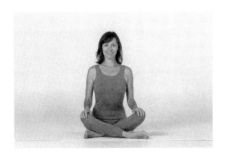

11. *Easy Sitting Twist, any version, 30-60 seconds each side*

12. *Easy Sitting Pose, version 1, 2 or 3, exhalation lengthening breath for 12 rounds*

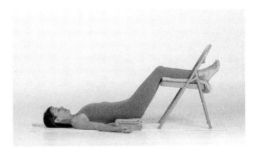

13. *Legs Up the Wall Pose, version 4, 5–10 minutes*

Brain and Nervous System Health

Our colleague Dr. Rammohan Rao is both a neuroscientist who studies Alzheimer's disease and a yoga teacher. Ram has a daily asana practice, which he varies as much as possible. He says he makes sure to include inverted poses because they calm the chattering of the mind and also "put our body in a position to take advantage of gravity to assist in the blood flow back toward the heart and head." (Studies have shown that aging is associated with reduced cerebral blood flow that can have deleterious health effects.) He also meditates to settle his unruly mind, practices pranayama to reduce stress, and uses the wisdom of yoga to cultivate contentment and maintain his mental health. He says:

> I incorporate yoga as part of my daily mental exercise regime. Yoga to me is not just about asanas but all forms of the discipline that bring the body-mind-breath in tune. I sincerely feel that my yoga practice is keeping me mentally agile as well as physically fit.[1]

About Your Brain and Nervous System

In the classic Steve Martin movie, *The Man with Two Brains*, Dr. Michael Hfuhruhurr visits the lab of mad scientist Dr. Necessiter, who has a collection of brains stored in glass jars, and falls in love with brain 21,

Anne Uumellmahaye, with whom he communicates telepathically. Well, yes, we loved that movie, but it's a perfect example of how not to think about the brain.

For some reason, most of us do tend to think about the brain the way it's portrayed in that movie—as a separate entity from the rest of the body where all cognition and emotion takes place (while the body does the work of keeping us alive).

But that's not really how it works. First of all, your brain plays an absolutely essential role in keeping your body alive. Through a network of nerves, your brain is connected to all of the other organs, structures, and systems of your body, and it actually keeps you breathing, keeps your heart beating, and coordinates all of the other functions, such as those of the digestive and immune systems that are keeping you healthy and active.

As for the thinking and feeling parts, our senses—sight, hearing, smell, taste, and touch (which is present in our entire skin)—are an essential part of how our brain interacts with and understands the world around us. So maybe your entire body is part of your brain! For example, the sensation you experience on the bottoms of your feet as you walk on an uneven surface is information your brain needs to keep you from falling.

This is why when we discuss yoga for brain health, it doesn't make sense to address the single organ—and its cognitive abilities—on its own. Instead, we will address your brain along with the entire nervous system that your brain uses to communicate with the rest of your body. Because your brain is a part of your body—just like your heart or liver—we will address how keeping your body itself healthy is as vital for maintaining brain health as is staying mentally and socially active.

Learning a bit about the basic components that make up the brain will help you understand how your yoga practice can have a stronger influence on the health of your brain than you might think.

About Your Brain

As you probably know, there are separate areas in your brain that provide specific functions. For example, the deeper parts of your brain manage background functions, such as digestion, blood pressure, and hormonal balance, and the more superficial parts control your conscious thoughts and actions. But throughout your life, your brain changes. This "neuroplasticity" allows your brain to grow and rewire itself in response to stimulation and learning. This is why brain-damaged stroke patients can relearn skills and why a healthy part of the brain can take over the function of a damaged part.

Your overall physical condition influences the health of your brain just as it does all of your organs. And maintaining adequate blood flow to and around your brain is essential for maintaining its structure and functioning. Your stress levels also influence your brain. Chronic stress can cause foggy thinking and, over longer periods of time, can even change the structure of your brain for the worse by shrinking certain areas. Finally, the amount of sleep you get affects your brain because in the short run too little sleep leaves you drowsy and unable to concentrate and in the long run it leads to impaired memory and physical performance. Some scientists even believe that sleep actually helps clear out toxins from your brain, which is vital for its long-term health.

The organ itself is connected to your spinal cord through the brainstem, which provides your brain with access to the nerves that control conscious movement, sensory input, and basic bodily functions, including heart rate and breathing. Although the brain and brainstem are protected by the blood-brain barrier, blood vessels surround the entire brain, so your circulatory system can deliver fuel to it and remove waste from it.

NERVOUS SYSTEM. Your brain communicates with your entire body through your central and peripheral nervous systems (see page 182).

GUT. Although your brain has two-way communication with every part of your body, it has a special two-way relationship with your gut. The human gut has a semi-independent nervous system called the "enteric nervous system," which is derived from the same embryonic neural crest cells that gave rise to the brain. Your gut is in constant communication with your brain, primarily through your central and peripheral nervous systems but also through neuropeptides to regulate complex feeding behavior and pain perception. And there is new evidence that even your gut microbiota (the friendly bacteria that reside in your gut) communicate with and coordinate signals between the gut and the brain. So keeping your gut happy and healthy will benefit your brain health as well.

OTHER SYSTEMS. Your circulatory system supplies fuel to and removes waste from your brain, which keeps it healthy. If the cardiovascular system is functioning less than optimally, for example, due to plaque buildup in the large blood vessels leading to the brain, or if it has weak spots that could rupture and bleed, your risk of having a stroke increases. So keeping your circulatory system healthy with yoga can contribute to maintaining brain health. Your immune system may also have a special relationship with your brain. A new theory about the origins of Alzheimer's disease points to a compromised immune system that leaves the brain vulnerable to infection. Fortunately, the same yoga practices you do for your heart and cardiovascular system will also support your immune system.

About Your Nervous System

Although we tend to think about our nervous systems only when we're feeling stressed (or nervous!), your nervous system is essential for your survival and provides the following necessary functions:

- Controls background processes that keep your body alive and healthy, such as breathing, maintaining normal temperature, and adjusting blood pressure to match activity
- Responds to external stimuli (perceived by your senses), such as having a positive reaction to a beautiful smell, a pain response to a burn, or a stress response to an oncoming car
- Obeys your conscious mental instructions, such as to talk, move, or breathe more slowly

By communicating through your nerves, your nervous system constantly monitors your body's internal activities and tries to keep all the systems in a healthy balance called "homeostasis." Your nervous system also monitors your external environment to assess if it is safe or dangerous and sends messages to your body either to relax and enjoy or act quickly to get to safety.

Your nervous system consists of two main parts: the central nervous system and the peripheral nervous system. However, even though we—and our anatomy books!—always discuss the central nervous system and peripheral nervous system as two separate systems, they really form one connected, continuous system that is in constant communication with all its components.

CENTRAL NERVOUS SYSTEM. Made up of your spinal cord and your brain, your central nervous system receives and processes information from all over your body. In response to conscious thoughts, your central nervous system sends nerve impulses to your peripheral nervous system to make requested actions happen. When your central nervous system receives nerve impulses from your senses and your autonomic nervous system (which keep your background systems in balance), it sends nerve impulses to make your body react appropriately.

Besides communicating through your nerves, your central nervous system also communicates with your organs and the rest of your body through chemical and hormonal messages. For example, the pituitary gland in your brain conveys information to other nerves and organs through the release of neurotransmitters or hormones.

PERIPHERAL NERVOUS SYSTEM. This system is made up of the nerves that connect your spinal cord to your entire musculoskeletal system (all of your muscles, bones, and joints) and to all of your internal organs except your brain. These nerves either deliver information to your central nervous system or receive instructions from it. For example, when you decide to raise your arms in Warrior 1 Pose, your brain sends a message via the peripheral nervous system to the appropriate muscles. When you're stressed, your peripheral nervous system speeds up your heart rate. Likewise, if you cut yourself, taste some chocolate, or sniff a flower, your peripheral nervous system lets your brain know all about it. The peripheral nervous system is made up of the somatic and autonomic systems.

Somatic Nervous System. This provides voluntary control of body movements. In yoga, we use our somatic nervous system when we practice poses, perform breath practices, stay still in meditation, and consciously relax muscles in restorative poses. Obviously we want our somatic nervous system to function optimally because to function well in our daily lives, we need quick and coordinated responses to our mental requests for movement or rest. Your senses are also connected to your brain through the somatic nervous system.

Autonomic Nervous System. This controls your body's involuntary functions, including your body temperature, your heartbeat and blood pressure, your breathing, your digestion, and your stress response. It's called "autonomic" because it works automatically without your conscious effort. (You don't need to tell your heart to beat like you tell your front knee to bend to 90 degrees in Warrior 2 Pose.) See chapter 9 for further information about the autonomic nervous system.

Aging and Your Brain and Nervous System

For most people, the age-related changes to the brain and nervous system that we will describe here occur gradually over time and typically result in only minimal loss of function, so many of us will not see a significant impact on our daily activities. Of course this is not true for everyone, and a growing percentage of much older people—such as those with certain genetic tendencies—do develop more serious conditions. Because these age-related conditions are serious, it makes good sense for all of us to take preventative measures. So let's take a closer look at how aging affects your brain and nervous system so you can better understand why yoga is so beneficial for fostering brain and nervous system health and know which practices will provide you with the appropriate benefits. In general, if you're practicing yoga for cardiovascular health as described in chapter 7, you're already doing a good job of fostering brain health, too.

BRAIN. With age, the brain tissue gradually shrinks a little, more in some areas then others. The neurons also gradually shrink (a few die off and are not replaced), and the connections between them are reduced. However, due to its neuroplasticity, your brain will also continue to grow, building new neurons and neural synapses, especially if you keep on learning and challenging your brain, and meditation practice will actually strengthen the brain itself.

The arteries that feed the brain gradually shrink and narrow as well, and the blood-brain barrier can become leaky, which together can, in some people, decrease the amount of blood and nutrition getting to the brain and reduce the ability to keep toxins out. However, you can improve blood flow and vessel health through aerobic exercise, including active yoga practices, as well as movements that improve circulation, such as inverted poses. In addition, maintaining good sleep habits can help clear toxins from your brain.

In some people, there is an increase in inflammation and the formation of toxic molecules called "free radicals," both of which can damage brain cells and lead to more cell death. But you can use stress management to prevent inflammation, as described in chapter 9. In addition, as you may have heard, tangles and plaques develop in the brains of some older adults. However, only about 10–20 percent of the people with these tangles and plaques go on to develop serious brain diseases, such as Alzheimer's and Parkinson's, and scientists are still unsure about the relationship between those diseases and the tangles and plaques. So for now, if you're concerned about serious brain diseases, focus on stress management, exercise, and good sleep.

For most people, the overall effect of these changes will be a modest decrease in brain function and a gradually worsening memory. The ability to perform tasks, learn new information or skills, and problem-solve may also slow down. But keep in mind that with practice older adults can improve at these and other cognitive tasks, including vocabulary, verbal knowledge, and information analysis. We also know that regular exercise, including an active asana practice, and stress management have overall beneficial effects on brain function and structure, as does regular meditation.

NERVES. The nerves of the central and peripheral nervous systems very gradually shrink with age, as does the insulation around them. Aging also reduces the blood flow to your nerves, decreasing the nourishment provided to and the waste collected from them. In a small percentage of people this causes the nerves to work less efficiently. You can maintain nerve health by supporting the health of your overall cardiovascular system, eating a healthy diet that keeps blood sugar at normal levels, and stretching your entire body to loosen muscles and fascia that can constrict nerves.

SPINAL CORD. The bones that enclose your spinal cord tend to gradually thin, and the cushioning between the bones tends to wear out, which for some people can result in arthritis of the spine, degenerating or bulging discs, and spinal fractures. You can help minimize these changes by fostering the strength and flexibility of your spine and by maintaining good posture.

PERIPHERAL NERVOUS SYSTEM. As a result of age-related changes, the nerves of your peripheral nervous system relay messages between your body and your brain a bit more slowly, causing your body to respond less rapidly and reducing your coordination, speed of movement, and the strength of your muscular responses. You can help minimize these changes with exercise, including an active yoga practice, to maintain overall strength, flexibility, balance, and agility.

The slowing of nerve transmission and aging itself can also affect your senses, leading to reduced or even lost sensory feedback, including diminished senses of touch, sight, hearing, smell, and taste, decreased proprioception, and changes in pain perception. Although many older adults have significant changes to vision and hearing, for almost everyone the amount of overall change to the other senses is modest. To compensate for any of these losses, working on strength, flexibility, and especially balance and agility can help you continue to move well through your everyday life.

In your autonomic nervous system, slightly slower nerve transmission can affect how well your brain communicates with the organs and systems whose functions it coordinates, including the cardiovascular system, the digestive system, and the urinary system. In a small percentage of people, this can lead to less efficient functioning of all of those systems, resulting in irregular heartbeats, sluggish digestion, or bladder problems. For these people, exercise, including active yoga practice, and stress management can improve the overall functioning of the autonomic nervous system.

HOW YOGA HELPS

Because your brain is connected to all the other organs, structures, and systems of your body, what we do to keep our other organs and systems healthy has an effect on our brains, and we shouldn't be surprised by that. But we are surprised! We tend to think we can keep the brain healthy just by feeding it new information and experiences, such as by learning new languages, playing music, and doing crossword puzzles. But physical exercise could be as or more important than mental exercise. In fact, a recent study that looked at both leg strength and cognitive ability in twins as they aged showed that those who maintained better leg strength as a result of exercising had better memory and other cognitive functions than their nonexercising twin.

Because yoga includes active exercise, resting poses, stress management practices, and equanimity practices that help you maintain overall physical and spiritual health, as well as ongoing opportunities for learning, it's surprisingly effective for brain health.

Exercising

Regular exercise leads to structural changes in your brain that improve cognition. It also increases nerve branching and in some cases triggers regeneration of nerve cells, especially in the brain's memory centers. Most importantly, this kind of exercise helps keep your cardiovascular system healthy. Your cardiovascular system has a large impact on your brain because the more blood that flows to your brain, the more oxygen and other important nutrients will reach it (this may partly explain the cognitive improvements associated with exercise). Also, because aging causes a decline in blood flow to the nerves, exercising to improve the blood flow to them will help maintain their health.

A regular, well-rounded asana practice provides an excellent form of exercise, fostering strength, flexibility, balance, and agility. But targeting cardiovascular health with your practice could be especially helpful for brain health. As our colleague Ram says, "What is good for the heart is good for the brain." (See chapter 7 for more information.)

NERVE HEALTH. Tight muscles and fascia due to a sedentary lifestyle, an active lifestyle that excludes stretching, or injuries that create scar tissue can compress your peripheral nerves. Static stretches and dynamic movements can help release tight areas and create space around the nerves, improving their health and ability to function.

You can also use your asana practice to support the health of your somatic nervous system by practicing a wide variety of poses and movement patterns to activate all those nerves on a regular basis and by practicing balance poses and flow sequences to keep your proprioceptors (the nerves that allow you to sense where you are in space) healthy. This will help counteract the age-related slowing of nerve messages to the muscles involved in conscious action, which affects coordination and speed of movement, as well as strength of muscle response.

SPINE HEALTH. Using your asana practice to maintain healthy posture and proper alignment of your spinal bones will help to keep your spinal cord safe from pinching and narrowing, which could cause nerve pain or dysfunction. And you can maintain the strength of the spinal bones themselves by practicing static poses, including backbends, forward bends, twists, and side bends, that move your spine in all directions.

Reducing Chronic Stress

While stress hormones initially sharpen your attention and spur you to take needed action, chronic stress can cause constant fear, worry, anxiety, and depression, which affect your ability to think clearly and reduce your ability to consider a wide variety of options. Chronic exposure to stress hormones also weakens blood vessels, kills off neurons, and shrinks the hippocampus, resulting in memory loss. Chronic stress also speeds up the normal aging of other cells that in turn affect the structure and function of your brain.

For brain and nervous system health, using any of the stress management techniques described in chapter 9 will help you dial down stress levels when you are suffering from chronic stress. You will not only create a mental state of calm with these practices, but you will also expand your thought-behavior repertoire to include a wider range of possibilities.

Reducing chronic stress also reduces inflammation, which can cause depression, anxiety, dementia, and even schizophrenia. Although we don't know for sure that you can prevent these conditions, you can help prevent inflammation in general by focusing on stress management.

Using your yoga practice to keep stress levels in check and manage your stress during challenging periods also supports the health of your nervous system overall. Spending more time in the rest-and-digest state (described in chapter 9) provides healing time for your nervous system as well as your brain. Managing chronic stress also reduces the risk of developing conditions that can negatively impact the nervous system (such as diabetes and hypertension).

Even if you're not experiencing chronic stress, it's beneficial for you to rest your brain and nervous system. Because restorative poses practiced with a mental focus and gentle inverted poses switch your nervous system to the rest-and-digest state and quiet your mind, they're perfect poses for resting your nervous system and your brain. During times of mental busyness or stress, a restful yoga practice can provide a healthy break during your day.

Sleep

For your brain and nervous system to function optimally and stay healthy, you need a good night's sleep. As we mentioned earlier, chronic sleep problems can have especially serious effects, such as impaired memory and accelerated mental decline, and may even be linked to dementia. They can also lead to hypertension and irregular heartbeat, causing poor blood flow into the brain and making you more susceptible to degenerative diseases or infections.

On the other hand, sleep triggers memory consolidation, which brings order to the chaos of information you received through your senses during your waking hours and preserves the organized information as memories. Studies show that people who slept well after learning a task do better when tested later than those who did not sleep well. Other studies show that good sleep stabilizes mood swings and helps regulate emotions.

Just as sleep gives your body time to heal, it allows neurons to lower their neurochemical activity and repair themselves (without sleep, neurons become "fatigued" and begin to malfunction). Sleep also helps to clear out toxins from the brain as well as from the body, reducing the risk of several brain diseases. Some scientists even think this is the real purpose of sleep!

Fortunately, yoga can be really helpful for improving sleep, and we provide tips for improving your sleep in chapter 9.

Brain Strength

Meditation has a special role to play in brain health. Not only does practicing meditation improve mental function, including your ability to focus and to maintain willpower, it literally strengthens your brain! Studies of longtime meditators show that these practitioners have more cortical folding (brain gyrification) than people who do not meditate. This additional folding may enable their brains to process information more quickly. See chapter 10 for information on meditation.

Learning

Just as physical exercise builds muscle strength, mental exercise tones thinking skills and memory. While aging results in the loss of some of our brain neurons, the ability of our brains to grow and change means that learning will actually cause our brain neurons to grow and existing neurons to be repurposed.

If you can remember back to your first yoga class, you will realize what a wonderful learning experience it was: All of those strange movements and body shapes and weird names for the poses, maybe even in a strange language. All of that talk about various muscles and bones you'd never thought about. And maybe there were even quotes from yoga texts that you'd never heard of before. For beginners, just learning about yoga provides great exercise for the brain. But even for longtime practitioners, yoga provides a wealth of opportunities for ongoing learning, including:

- Trying new poses, variations of poses you already know, or different ways of propping
- Trying new practices, such as mudras, breath practices, or meditation techniques
- Exploring different yoga traditions by taking classes from different teachers
- Studying yoga philosophy and history
- Learning Sanskrit

Community

Staying socially active as you age provides several important benefits for brain health, including reducing the risk of depression and delaying the onset of dementia. Because being socially active requires that you plan, participate, and be attentive and alert, it qualifies as mental exercise, helping build healthy brain cells and the connections between them.

Being part of the yoga community provides you with a lifelong connection to like-minded people, as there are always other people to practice with no matter how old you are. Going regularly to classes helps you stay in touch with yoga friends, but not everyone can afford paying for frequent classes. Our techniques section below includes several recommendations for different ways to participate in the yoga community.

Equanimity and Brain Health

Have you ever tried to think straight when you're depressed, anxious, or angry? Cultivating equanimity is a powerful way to help you think more clearly and make better decisions overall. All the equanimity practices that we recommend in chapter 10 can help you stay emotionally balanced and clear-headed. Try as many different practices as you can to see which work best for you.

Nutrition

Good nutrition is as important for your brain as it is for your heart and cardiovascular health. Eating a healthy, nutritious diet fuels your brain and nervous system and helps support their health. And because your gut is connected to your brain, keeping it healthy and happy by maintaining a good diet also benefits your brain and nervous system health. Although it's beyond the scope of this book to go into the topic in detail, we have some suggestions in chapter 9 on using yoga to support healthy eating.

USING YOGA FOR BRAIN AND NERVOUS SYSTEM HEALTH

This section provides information on how to use your yoga practice to foster brain health as well as central and peripheral nervous system health. If you are already practicing well-rounded active sequences that include a few restorative poses (or at the least a long Relaxation Pose), breath work, and meditation, you're off to a great start—regular exercise, stress management, and meditation for brain strength are all going to help your brain and your nervous system. For those who want to focus especially on brain and/or nervous system health—whether you are concerned about brain health in general or have a family history of brain problems, such as early onset dementia or Parkinson's disease—the following section provides recommendations for targeting these areas.

Techniques for Fostering Brain and Nervous System Health

WHAT TO PRACTICE. For your balanced practices that include asanas, stress management, and meditation, be sure to vary the sequences that you practice as well as the individual poses that you include to keep your sessions fresh and stimulating for your brain! On rest days consider practicing a short "brain practice," which could be meditation, a yoga philosophy study session on your own or with friends, or even time spent reading yoga books to find new poses, practices, and sequences to try.

HOW OFTEN TO PRACTICE. In general, work toward practicing five to six days a week. Because exercise is important for brain health, we recommend practicing an active asana sequence (or another type of exercise, such as walking) three to four days a week. On the other days, either do your short brain-stimulating practice, an equanimity practice of your choice, or—if chronic stress is a problem—a short stress management session (see below).

STATIC POSES. The more physically challenging a pose is, the greater the workload on your heart, and exercising your cardiovascular system is a particularly good way to foster brain as well as heart health. So we recommend including the same challenging poses in your sequences for brain health as you include for cardiovascular health. See chapter 7 for pose recommendations and timings.

Besides providing exercise to benefit your brain and nervous system, static poses stretch your tissues, including the tissue around your nerves. With a regular asana practice, you can release holding patterns around your nerves, permitting more slide and glide through muscles and joints, which allows them to function more effectively.

Finally, balance poses help improve your proprioception, fostering the health of the specialized nerves that allow you to sense where your body is in space. To add learning into your asanas, vary your static poses as much as possible. Switch which side you start on, change your arm positions, or create a new version of a familiar pose.

DYNAMIC POSES. Dynamic poses and flow sequences practiced for their cardiovascular benefits also foster brain health. So we recommend including the same dynamic poses in your sequences for brain health as you would for cardiovascular health. See chapter 7 for recommendations for dynamic poses to practice and how fast to move between poses.

Like static poses, dynamic poses stretch tissues, including those around the nerves, so you can use them to release holding patterns around your nerves, allowing them to function more effectively. Also, because you are moving quickly from one position to another, all dynamic poses and flow sequences improve the functioning of your proprioceptors.

To add learning into your practices, vary your dynamic poses and flow sequences as much as possible and experiment with inventing new ones.

MEDITATION. If you already have a regular meditation practice, simply continue practicing as usual. If you do not currently meditate, we strongly recommend that you start because meditation has been shown to improve brain structure and function. See chapter 10 for information.

STRESS MANAGEMENT. When you're not feeling particularly stressed out, a well-rounded practice that includes active asanas and short sessions of a stress management technique of your choice will help keep your stress levels in check. If you choose to meditate every day or do breath practices, restorative yoga, or supported inversions on your rest days, all the better. However, because stress management is so important for brain health, if you're experiencing chronic stress or entering a stressful period in your life, we recommend practicing at least a short stress management session for about twenty minutes every day. What you practice for stress management could be any of the relaxation practices you prefer or that work in your particular circumstances (see chapter 9 for more information).

EQUANIMITY. Because cultivating equanimity as you age will allow you to think more clearly and make better decisions as well as help you handle any changes to your life and circumstances that arise, we recommend incorporating equanimity practices into your daily life. See chapter 10 for ideas.

SLEEP. If chronic insomnia is a problem for you, we strongly recommend that you use your yoga practice to support better sleep (see chapter 9). Even though relaxing while you're awake may seem counterintuitive if you just want to go to sleep, we urge you to do this important work as the payoffs are worth it.

LEARNING. Because your brain is "plastic" and continues to actively grow and rewire itself when it is stimulated, we recommend using your yoga practice as a way to keep learning. Try new poses or new variations of familiar poses, new sequences, and new practices beyond asanas (such as mudras or breath practices) on a regular basis. We also recommend studying yoga philosophy because in addition to helping you learn to cultivate equanimity, this will expose you to new concepts and terminology. And because learning a new language is especially effective for brain health, try working on your Sanskrit!

COMMUNITY. Remaining socially active supports brain health and delays the onset of dementia. Attending yoga classes and participating in your local yoga community is a good way to stay socially active as well as to keep your practice going strong. If you're not already active in the yoga community, there are many ways to join:

- Find a regular class you can afford
- Attend free events at your local yoga studio
- Go on a retreat (if it's in your budget)
- Attend yoga conferences
- Practice yoga with a friend
- Attend yoga book groups
- Participate in an online yoga community
- Volunteer for yoga community service
- Plan your own yoga event

BRAIN HEALTH PRACTICE

This sequence includes a well-balanced set of poses for fostering brain health, including active poses to provide all-around exercise and inverted poses to improve circulation and lower stress levels. It also includes meditation for improving brain strength and special tasks and variations (learning pose names or practicing with closed eyes) for mental challenges.

Although the sequence itself will help improve brain health, if you wish, you can include some additional mental exercises. As you start in Hero Pose, choose a sutra from Patanjali's Yoga Sutras and read it aloud in Sanskrit three times and then read the English translation aloud three times in a row. Then, in the final pose of the sequence, recall the sutra and use the translation as a mantra for your meditation session, repeating it mentally as you breathe comfortably. In addition, we have included the Sanskrit names for the poses in the sequence. If you're not already familiar with them, say each one aloud as you practice each pose.

When you practice the Sun Salutations, do the first round with your eyes open. Then do two to four more rounds with your eyes closed. For your asymmetrical poses, if you are used to doing your right side first, switch to the left first for this sequence. (Of course, if you usually start to the left, you should switch to the right.)

For photos that illustrate the individual movements in the Sun Salutation, see the "Dynamic Poses and Flow Sequences" section on page 282.

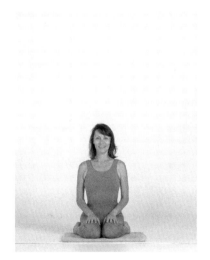

1. Hero Pose (Virasana), any version, 1–2 minutes

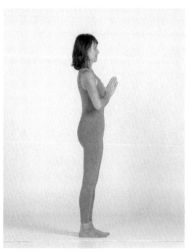

2. Mini Sun Salutations (Surya Namaskar), 3–5 rounds

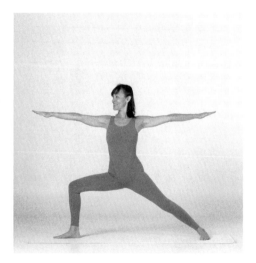

3. Warrior 2 Pose (Virabradrasana 2), any version, 30–60 seconds each side

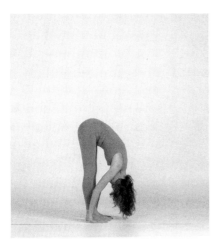

4. Standing Forward Bend (Uttanasana), version 1, 1 minute

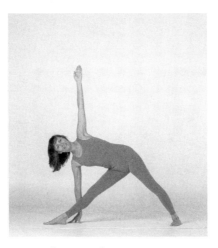

5. Triangle Pose (Trikonasana), any version, 30–60 seconds each side

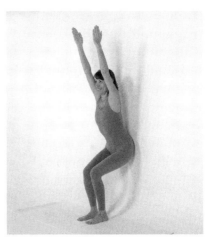

6. Powerful Pose (Utkatasana), version 3, 30 seconds, 2 times

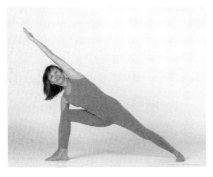

7. Extended Side Angle Pose (Utthita Parsva-konasana), any version, 30–60 seconds each side

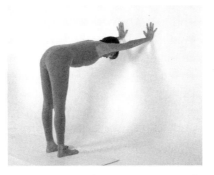

8. Half Downward-Facing Dog Pose (Arda Adho Mukha Svanasana), any version you don't normally do, 30–60 seconds

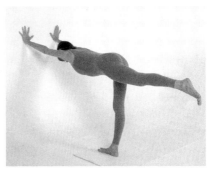

9. Warrior 3 Vinyasa (Virabradrasana 3), 3–6 times on first side, 3–6 times on second side

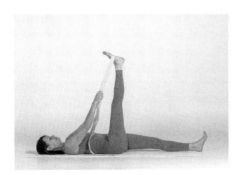

10. Reclined Leg Stretch (Supta Padan-gusthasana), version 1, 1–2 minutes each side

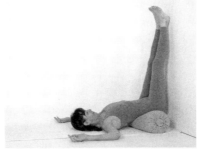

11. Legs Up the Wall Pose (Viparita Karani), 5–10 minutes. Choose a version you don't normally do and vary your arms

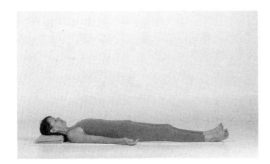

12. Relaxation Pose (Savasana), version 2, 5–10 minutes

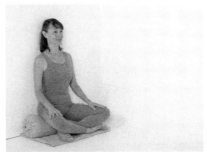

13. Easy Sitting Pose (Sukasana), version 3, 3–5 minutes. Use sutra for meditation

9

Stress Management

WHEN TOM, A VETERAN LANCE CORPORAL IN THE MARINE CORPS, was introduced to yoga, his marriage of twenty-nine years was coming to an end and his life was falling apart. Although he'd been out of the Corps for several decades, he'd never dealt with the issues that came up during his service. He felt he just couldn't cope anymore and started planning his suicide. But instead of immediately going through with those plans, he went to someone he trusted, which led to a ten-day stay in an acute care unit followed by a six-week inpatient PTSD program at a local VA hospital. It was during the PTSD program that Tom was introduced to yoga. He was still feeling suicidal, so when he learned that there was going to be a yoga retreat for veterans sponsored by the Veterans Yoga Project, he decided to go as part of his treatment. He said that the light came on for him during the first yoga session at the retreat when he discovered that there was so much more to yoga than just stretching:

> The mindfulness practices taught during yoga both at the retreat and in the program helped me find a way to break the loops running through my head. It allowed me to take a breath or two and stop thinking too much. It showed me how to have an emotion without letting that emotion rule me and my actions.[1]

The Veterans Yoga Project did another life-changing thing for Tom, who had not slept more than an hour or two at a time for five years: it enabled him to get a full eight hours of sleep a night. Tom says that at the retreat he learned how to quiet his mind and let things go without holding on, which finally allowed him to sleep. He still practices the techniques that he learned there to this day.

Stress has a pretty bad reputation these days, but without at least a little bit of stress in your system, you'd pass out when you tried to get out of bed in the morning! So some amount of stress is important for your survival. On the other hand, yes, too much stress for a long period of time is truly dangerous for your physical, mental, and emotional health. And because how you adapt and respond to stress is considered one of the seven pillars of aging, practicing stress management could very well have an effect on how you age.

Maintaining a good balance between stress and relaxation is what you should really be aiming for. Mostly that means reducing chronic stress levels because, as you might imagine, there aren't many people out there who are too relaxed. To help you understand what it means to balance stress and relaxation (and determine when you need one or the other), let's take a closer look at your autonomic nervous system.

Your Autonomic Nervous System

Let's say you're sitting outside in the garden talking with a friend, and you're feeling very comfortable and relaxed. Then your friend tells you about an interesting idea he has, and you suddenly perk up a bit. You then pitch in with an idea of your own and that leads to an animated discussion. What's happening here? Are you relaxed or stressed? Is it possible that you are both at the same time?

Ding, ding, ding! Yes, it's both at the same time. As we described in chapter 8, your autonomic nervous system, which controls background processes that keep your body alive and healthy, such as breathing, maintaining normal temperature, and adjusting blood pressure to match activity, is divided into two subsystems: the sympathetic and parasympathetic nervous systems. Understanding how these two subsystems work together to provide you with a healthy balance of activity and relaxation will help you learn how to use your yoga practice to bring yourself into balance. We'll look first at the sympathetic nervous system and follow that with the parasympathetic nervous system.

Your Sympathetic Nervous System

Let's say one night you're driving your car down a dark, winding road through a forest when suddenly a deer bolts into the road. Your heart begins to pound and your breath speeds up as you quickly try to take evasive action. Is this stress? On another night, you're meeting someone you've just started dating. When you spot them on the street coming toward you, your heart begins to pound and your breath speeds up. It feels kind of like stress, but in a good way—exciting. What's going on here?

Your sympathetic system stimulates you when you need to be active. The activity can be as basic as getting out of bed in the morning, writing an e-mail, or practicing gentle yoga poses, something more challenging, such as running a race or giving a public talk, or something life threatening such as trying to avoid a car accident.

STRESS RESPONSE. By activating your stress response, your sympathetic nervous system prepares your body and mind for action, stimulating your heart to beat faster and stronger, slightly raising your blood pressure to improve blood flow, opening your airways so you can breathe more easily, and stimulating your thought processes so you can assess your situation and think more quickly.

The term "stress response" describes the response of your mind and body when you are faced with *any* challenge. Sometimes the response is to a real or perceived threat, from serious life or death situations to frustrating situations like doing your taxes or getting lost. Other times the response is to a positive challenge, such as running a race, falling in love, brainstorming ideas, or creating a work of art.

The strength of your response corresponds to the amount of excitement, disorientation, discomfort, anger, or fear that you are feeling. If you're only mildly chilly or arriving in a new country for the first time, you probably won't react with an intense stress response. However, if the stressor is something that requires a strong response, such as feeling an earthquake or even imagining for a moment that the washing machine shaking the house is an earthquake, your stress response will be much stronger.

FIGHT-OR-FLIGHT STATE. In extreme situations—where serious action is needed—your sympathetic nervous system triggers the fight-or-flight response. In this state, generally you actually are in danger, threatened, or think you are in danger. For example, if you are about to get into a car accident, your nervous system sends quick signals to your adrenal glands to release adrenaline, unleashing a rapid physical response designed to get you to safety. In this state, your sympathetic nervous system curbs nourishment, restoration, and healing functions because they will slow you down. Being in the fight-or-flight state is normal and healthy as long as it doesn't happen too frequently or continue for a long period of time, which is when it becomes chronic stress. See "Understanding Stress" on page 132 for more information.

Your Parasympathetic Nervous System

Your parasympathetic nervous system is responsible for nourishing, restoring, and healing your body and mind. As you move through your day, whether you are totally relaxed, slightly active, or very active, your parasympathetic nervous system stimulates digestion, activates various metabolic processes, and keeps your immune system working efficiently.

Now imagine that you're lying on a beautiful beach, feeling the warmth of the sun on your skin and listening to the sound of waves lapping at the shore, and you're feeling totally comfortable and relaxed. What is happening to you?

Another time you're sitting alone in your house, meditating on your breath. Your knee hurts a bit, your thoughts seem wild, and you feel fidgety and restless. But you keep coming back to your breath, and after several minutes your mind begins to settle and quiet down. What's happening to you now? How is this different from being on the beach?

RELAXATION RESPONSE. Your parasympathetic nervous system responds to safe circumstances or a secure environment by activating the relaxation response, causing your heart and breath rate to slow, your blood pressure to drop, your energy use to decrease, and your digestion and immune systems to function optimally. If you successfully avoided the car crash in our earlier example, your system might slowly shift from the flight-or-flight state to the relaxation response once you got home and had some time to decompress.

You can trigger the relaxation response through conscious relaxation techniques (see below) or just by ordinary resting and relaxing while you are awake, such as listening to calming music or lying on a beach feeling the sun on your skin and hearing the waves. This is in contrast to activities that are distracting rather than relaxing. For example, while TV distracts us from our real-life concerns, it is not actually relaxing your nervous system because the action you're watching is typically very stimulating—as anyone who tries to go to bed after a scary movie or violent show soon realizes. The state of relaxation is also very different than sleep, providing a few different benefits. See "Understanding Conscious Relaxation and the Rest-and-Digest State" below for a comparison between relaxation and sleep.

CONSCIOUS RELAXATION. This term describes any technique you use to intentionally trigger the relaxation response, including meditation, breath practices that are calming, guided relaxation practices, and even gentle and restorative yoga asanas practiced mindfully. But the awesome thing about conscious relaxation is that you can use it anytime and anywhere—you don't need to fly to Hawaii. Although a quiet, peaceful environment is helpful, you can meditate or do breath practices in challenging environments, such as airports or waiting rooms.

REST-AND-DIGEST STATE. When you are physically still and your mind is quiet, your parasympathetic system functions optimally. In the rest-and-digest state, you are mentally and physically relaxed, your body's vital signs are in their calm state, and your immune, repair, and digestive systems are functioning optimally.

Being in the rest-and-digest state is normal and very desirable, as it gives your body and mind time to relax completely and recover from stressful periods. There's really no downside to spending a lot of time in this state, except that you probably wouldn't get very much done! You enter this state naturally when relaxing at home or out in nature or when you use conscious relaxation to trigger the relaxation response.

On an average day, when you're feeling rested and cheerful and are involved in normal work and social activities, your sympathetic and parasympathetic systems work together to keep you in balance, allowing you to be fully functional, stay healthy, and interact well with others. A well-balanced yoga practice, including both physical exercise and stress management practices, will help you maintain this balance when there are minor challenges in your life. It is only when you spend too much time with an overactive sympathetic nervous system resulting from ongoing stressful life circumstances that you can become out of balance. At this point, it's very important to take steps to reduce your chronic stress and bring yourself back into balance again. Chronic stress is harmful to your physical, emotional, and mental health, and conscious relaxation with yoga is the answer! (See "Understanding Conscious Relaxation and the Rest-and-Digest State" on page 135 for more information about relaxation.)

UNDERSTANDING STRESS

A wide range of experiences have the potential to cause us to experience a stress response, including physical discomfort, such as pain or cold, and psychological discomfort, such as being angry with someone or afraid of danger. A stressor can be something external, such as traveling to a foreign country or a car running a red light. It can also be internal, such as the fear of running out of money or an intense emotion that has the potential to change your life, such as falling in love.

Because you might need to fight or run, your sympathetic nervous system releases hormones (adrenaline, noradrenaline, and cortisol) to increase your heart rate, your blood pressure, and the blood flow to your muscles. It also dilates your airways to allow you to take deeper breaths, increases your muscle strength, and releases energy that your body has stored for emergencies. Because your body is working extra hard during stressful periods, if stress becomes more than just an occasional brief response to a serious threat, your body will wear out faster, which is one reason why heart disease is associated with chronic stress.

The sympathetic nervous system also affects your thinking, causing your mind to race to increase your ability to assess your current situation and make important decisions. It also narrows the scope of your thoughts to fight-or-flight possibilities. While the fight-or-flight mind helps you focus in an emergency, having a racing mind all the time causes emotional problems, such as anxiety and depression, as well as insomnia because you can't let go of your thoughts and fall asleep.

While your sympathetic nervous system is stimulating a fight-or-flight response, it is also slowing processes that you don't need during emergencies, such as digestion, urination, healing, and the restoration and building of tissues. So you can see why you don't want to be in a state of stress 24/7!

When you are stressed, try to step back and observe your physical sensations. Is your heart pounding? Are you nauseated? Is your mouth dry? Are your thoughts racing? Learn to notice when you're in this state so you can calm yourself if appropriate.

Acute Stress

Acute stress is a short-lived episode that triggers a natural, healthy response to danger, a perceived threat, or a physical challenge. This is something we can't and shouldn't eliminate from our lives. We all need to get out of danger sometimes, whether it's avoiding an oncoming car or protecting a family member from a threat. Our stress response also prepares us for some really good things in life, including running a race, brainstorming with a colleague, falling in love with someone, and even having an orgasm.

However, there are some times when an acute stress response might not be appropriate to the current situation, such as when your buttons are pushed during a family disagreement or in a traffic jam. In these cases, you can use simple breath awareness or calming breath practices to dial your response down to be in line with the situation.

Chronic Stress

Chronic stress is ongoing stress that never lets up. Many different life circumstances can cause chronic stress, from job pressures, marriage or family problems, and financial or health problems to living in a stressful environment, such as a dangerous neighborhood or war zone. When your nervous system is continuously on the alert, your body and mind never have a chance to recover and recuperate, and they become overtaxed and can start to degrade. Some of the serious health problems chronic stress can contribute to include heart disease, high blood pressure, insomnia, fatigue, digestive disorders, headaches, chronic anxiety or depression, and a weakened immune system. That's why using yoga to reduce chronic stress helps prevent major age-related diseases as well as depression, anxiety, insomnia, obesity, and digestive problems, and promotes overall health by bolstering your immune system and reducing inflammation.

Sometimes you can change your circumstances to less stressful ones, and your yoga practice can help support you through those changes. Other times circumstances are beyond your control and yoga's stress management practices can help you face difficult challenges while at the same dialing down your stress levels.

MOODS AND EMOTIONAL DISORDERS. In general, chronic stress has a negative effect on your moods. When your sympathetic nervous system is overstimulated, you may experience any of the following negative feelings: anxiety, restlessness, irritability, anger, sadness, and depression. These moods are not only unpleasant but can also interfere with your ability to conduct yourself in a way that is in line with your values and goals. For example, if you're restless and irritated, it's hard to be patient with and loving to family members and friends.

In people who are susceptible, full-blown anxiety or depression may even develop. There are several different theories about the mechanisms that cause depression and anxiety. One is that chronic stress leads to elevated hormones, such as the stress hormone cortisol, and reduced serotonin and other neurotransmitters in the brain, including dopamine, all of which are associated with depression. Another recent theory is that depression may be caused by inflammation, which itself can be triggered by chronic stress. Even though research is still ongoing, the bottom line is that chronic stress can contribute to a whole range of emotional problems, so reducing it is an important aspect of preserving your emotional health.

CHRONIC STRESS AND YOUR THOUGHTS. The fight-or-flight state affects your thoughts as well as your feelings. Because you need to focus on solving the problem at hand, your thoughts narrow and become limited to fight-or-flight strategies. But when you are calmer, your thoughts are more expansive, allowing you to consider a much wider range of options, including more altruistic possibilities. You're also more able to feel empathy for others and connect and communicate with them more effectively.

Living with chronically high stress levels can have a negative impact on your thoughts. For example, a very strong stress response with only thoughts of fighting or running is appropriate for a soldier in an actual battle. But that same strong response and accompanying thoughts are not appropriate if that soldier is stuck in a traffic jam or working at an office.

Practicing stress management on a regular basis allows you to respond more appropriately to your situation. When your stress response is "optimum" for your situation, it's possible for you to consider options in line with your basic values and goals. Here's how Dan Libby, psychologist and founder of the Veterans Yoga Project, puts it:

> The basic gist is that regulating our autonomic nervous system, which really means activating the more newly evolved part of the parasympathetic nervous system via the vagus nerve, allows for an expansion of your thought-behavior repertoire. Instead of having a limited, narrow, tunnel vision, like we do when our sympathetic nervous system is dominant, we have more cognitive and behavioral options available to navigate our world.[2]

Obviously being able to live in line with your basic values and goals is going to contribute to your equanimity. You'll be able to interact well with other people and solve problems in a more peaceful and productive way. Reducing chronic stress will help you keep your thought-behavior repertoire appropriate to your circumstances.

CHRONIC STRESS AND SLEEP. One of the common effects of an overactive sympathetic nervous system is insomnia. Your nervous system keeps you on the alert—and awake—so you're prepared to face imminent danger. But when your worries are about everyday life, staying awake in the middle of the night is counterproductive, as lack of sleep leaves you tired and unable to concentrate and deal effectively with your problems. If sleep deprivation continues, you can even develop impaired memory and mood swings.

Sleep is also necessary for your nervous system to work properly. Just as it gives your body time to heal itself, sleep also allows neurons to repair themselves. Without sleep, neurons become "fatigued" and begin to malfunction.

If sleep is a problem for you, it's a really good idea to consciously manage your daytime stress levels so that you don't go to bed with an overactive nervous system—this will improve your nights as well as your days. See "Yoga for Better Sleep" on page 155 for more information.

Understanding Conscious Relaxation and the Rest-and-Digest State

When you're in the rest-and-digest state, your nervous system is helping you recover from stressful periods. Because your body needs to rest and acquire new energy, it reduces the levels of stress hormones in your body, slowing your heart rate, decreasing your blood pressure, and so on. It also stimulates your digestive system, allowing it to function optimally and provide needed resources to your body. Resources that were directed to support fighting or running are now directed to support healing and immune system functions. When you're mildly stressed, your digestive, repair, and immune systems are still functioning fairly efficiently. However, they only function optimally when you're in the rest-and-digest state, so it is vital for you to spend some time in this state so you can rest, recover, and acquire energy.

The rest-and-digest state provides vital renewal for your mind as well as your body. In this state, you'll experience feelings of relaxation, as your racing mind slows down and your thoughts expand to consider a wide range of possibilities and observations.

Now you might be wondering whether you can't get the same results by taking a nap or by sleeping in on Sunday morning. A basic comparison with sleep will help you understand why it's not enough to just take a nap or drop into bed after a hard day.

Dreams. Dreams can actually cause stress because you may have nightmares or anxiety dreams. On the other hand, in the rest-and-digest state, the production of stress hormones and your stress-related symptoms—including both the physical and emotional ones—gradually decrease.

Oxygen Consumption. During sleep, your oxygen consumption decreases only 8 percent after about 4 or 5 hours. On the other hand, in the rest-and-digest state, oxygen consumption decreases rapidly to 10 to 20 percent during the first 3 minutes. When you are resting deeply, you need much less oxygen because you are not preparing to become active.

Blood Lactate. Blood lactate is a substance associated with anxiety attacks. In the rest-and-digest state, your blood lactate levels fall rapidly during the first 10 minutes. While you relax, your thoughts stop racing and your mind quiets while your body is resting and digesting. Sleep does not have the same effects on blood lactate levels.

Brain Waves. In the rest-and-digest state, alpha waves (slow brain waves) increase in intensity and frequency. Alpha waves are associated with relaxation and peacefulness. On the other hand, during sleep, your brain waves are quite different.

Dr. Roger Cole, a sleep researcher and longtime yoga teacher, says that during rest or meditation our brain waves may slow to the alpha rhythm (eight to twelve cycles per second), during which we remain quietly aware of ourselves and our surroundings without a lot of "self-directed mental processing." Sometimes they may slow even further to the theta rhythm (four to seven cycles per second), during which we may experience a sensation of floating, mental images like those in dreams, and withdrawal from the outside world. Although much is unknown about these unusual states, we do know that regular practice of conscious relaxation helps foster ongoing feelings of serenity, contentment, and even happiness.

How Yoga Helps with Stress

Because your autonomic nervous system responds to information it receives from your body and is also influenced by your state of mind, you can intentionally trigger the relaxation response. Yoga is a particularly effective way to do this because it provides such a wide range of options that you're sure to find at least one that works well for you.

The seven yoga tools we recommend all provide you with the ability to switch your nervous system from fight or flight to rest and digest. These stress management tools are not all interchangeable, however. Although you can use any of these practices to trigger the relaxation response, these

As I transitioned out of the military, yoga became more about balancing stress. Being a combat veteran, coming from environments that are heavily impacted by violence, it really allowed me to turn inward constructively, and that was such a powerful practice to be able to bridge the physical, mental, and emotional all together. I have been doing it ever since.

—John, US Navy

practices each have different roles to play in a balanced yoga practice. So let's compare and contrast them a bit.

Breath Practices (Pranayama)

Breath awareness provides a simple way to trigger the relaxation response. You can use it to quiet your nervous system or as a form of meditation. In addition, changing your breathing patterns provides you with a key to your nervous system, allowing you to calm, stimulate, or balance yourself. Practices that slow your breath or lengthen your exhalations are calming to your nervous system, so they are especially useful for both acute and chronic stress. For acute stress, lengthening your exhalation can help you in the moment to dial down an inappropriately strong response. For chronic stress, slowing your breath or lengthening your exhalation allows you to spend quality time in the rest-and-digest state. See "How to Practice Breath Awareness" on page 146 and "Breath Practices for Equanimity" on page 170 for instructions on breath practices.

Like meditation, pranayama is also an important component of classical yoga and precedes meditation as one of eight steps on the path to *samadhi* (union with the divine). It is considered an instrument to "steady the mind" and a gateway to *dharana* (concentration, which is the first phase of meditation).

Meditation

Meditation—which typically involves concentrating on a nonstressful sight, sound, or physical sensation—helps you to quiet your mind, which in turn switches your nervous system to the rest-and-digest state. All it takes is the following:

- A focus for your mind, such as a sound, word, phrase, physical sensation (your breath or your back resting on the floor or against a chair), or a fixed gaze on an object
- A nonjudgmental attitude about your performance
- Ten to twenty minutes

Options include both seated and reclined meditation. In addition, your asana practice can be a "moving meditation," as long as you have a focus for your mind (such as the physical sensations of your body in the pose) and an attitude of nonjudgment (refraining from judging how you look, how "well" you do the pose, or whether you're doing it "right").

The role of meditation in a balanced yoga practice is particularly important. Although you can use meditation for stress reduction, its role in classical yoga is to quiet the mind to allow union with the divine or liberation. It is also a powerful tool for studying your mind and slowly gaining more control over it. See chapter 10 for information on meditation and practicing yoga mindfully.

Restorative Yoga

Practicing relaxing or quieting yoga poses, such as restorative poses and supported forward bends, in a warm room will send a message to your nervous system that you're safe and comfortable. These modern yoga poses provide deep physical relaxation by supporting and relaxing your body and can trigger the relaxation response if you practice them with a mental focus. Classic examples are Reclined Cobbler's Pose and Supported Child's Pose.

Supported Inverted Poses

These poses use gravity to trigger the relaxation response through the mechanisms that control your blood pressure. As long as you are warm, quiet, and comfortable in the pose, all you have to do is let the pose work its magic. You don't need a mental focus to reach the rest-and-digest state, but without one you are not training your mind.

Relaxation Pose (Savasana)

In both classic and supported forms, Relaxation Pose, like restorative yoga poses, provides deep physical relaxation for your body and can trigger the relaxation response. Savasana is an ancient yoga pose and based on what we've read about the original practice, we feel that it is a reclining form of meditation. For some traditional yogis, it was a meditation on death—hence the literal translation, "Corpse Pose"—and it was sometimes even practiced alongside actual corpses. To practice Savasana properly, however, you must actually do the work of meditating while you are in the pose (and make sure you don't fall asleep). If you don't meditate while in Savasana, you are simply relaxing, which is okay if it is what you're after.

Guided Relaxation

Modern guided relaxation practices allow you to achieve physical relaxation and reduce stress levels by leading you through a deep physical relaxation experience and providing mental imagery to anchor you in the present moment. These include basic body scans and visualization practices, as well as formal practices such as *yoga nidra* (yogic sleep). Guided relaxation practices are specifically designed as relaxation techniques and do not replace meditation or pranayama in a balanced yoga practice. This is true of any form of Relaxation Pose in which an external voice is providing instructions and/or imagery for you. This book does not contain information about how to practice guided relaxation, but if it interests you, we recommend that you seek out some recordings.

Asanas

If you are feeling restless after being sedentary, an active asana practice can release physical stress from your body and burn off some of your pent-up energy, making it easier for you to practice meditation, breath practices, quieting yoga poses, or any other form of relaxation. Examples of active sequences in our book that will help prepare you for relaxation include our Cardiovascular Health, Easy Agility, and Lower Body Strength practices. You can also use your asana practice as a form of moving meditation by practicing mindfully as described in chapter 10. But either way, an active yoga practice is most effective for stress management if you finish with a short session of relaxation and/or meditation for at least ten minutes.

USING YOGA FOR STRESS

A well-rounded yoga practice that includes active asanas and short sessions of stress management will help keep your daily stress levels in check. If you meditate every day or do breath practices, restorative yoga, and/or supported inversions on your rest days, all the better.

However, the nature of human existence is such that we all go through times when our stress levels are higher than "normal," so this section provides techniques for handling periods of chronic stress.

Techniques for Managing Stress

HOW OFTEN TO PRACTICE. Although we don't recommend practicing a full-length active asana sequence seven days a week (your body periodically needs time to rest and recover), if you are going through a stressful period, we do recommend practicing at least a short stress management session for about twenty minutes every day. What you practice for these sessions could be any of the relaxation practices you prefer or that work for you: seated or reclined meditation, calming breath practices, one or two restorative and/or supported inverted poses, or a guided relaxation program. Because exercise is also important for reducing stress, you should aim to do an active asana practice (or another type of exercise, such as walking) three to four days a week.

HOW LONG TO PRACTICE. For a balanced asana session, such as one of our strength or flexibility sequences, we recommend practicing for thirty to forty-five minutes. For a short stress management session, we suggest you practice twenty minutes per day. You can actually divide these sessions up and practice one part in the morning and the other part later in the day. For example, you could practice active poses in the morning and restorative poses at the end of the day, or you could meditate for ten minutes in the morning and ten minutes in the evening.

WHAT TO PRACTICE. For days when you want to do a full-length active practice, use any sequence that includes a combination of poses for cultivating the four essential skills (strength, flexibility, balance, and agility) or a sequence that focuses on one of the skills. Generally, it makes sense to include the active poses at the beginning of your sequence, but if you're fatigued you can start with a resting pose and ease into the more active ones. Always quiet yourself down after the active poses with a stress management practice. For days when you just need a short stress management session, use a single practice or a combination of several practices that work for you in your particular circumstances.

STATIC POSES. These poses are good for grounding you when you're feeling anxious or flighty and for tiring yourself out a bit when you're feeling hyper. Standing poses, such as Warrior 2 Pose and Triangle Pose, are particularly effective. But a balanced practice that includes static poses from every category will engage your body and mind and release physical tension from your body. Practice mindfully for best results.

DYNAMIC POSES. Like static poses, dynamic poses engage your mind and release physical tension from your body. They can also mildly energize you when stress makes you feel fatigued. Be careful, however, not to practice (or breathe) too quickly, as this can overstimulate you. Again, for best results, practice mindfully.

SUPPORTED INVERTED POSES. For many people, supported inverted poses are so effective for calming the nervous system and quieting the mind that even just one fifteen-minute session of Legs Up the Wall Pose can turn the day around. If these poses work well for you, always include one or more near the end of your active practices. Choose poses that you can hold for extended periods of time and use appropriate propping to ensure that you'll be comfortable. Warming up for these poses with active or reclining poses that stretch your legs and open your shoulders may help you be less fidgety.

RESTORATIVE POSES. If stress is making you feel exhausted and depleted, you can put together an entire asana practice of restorative poses or even practice a single pose on its own. If you are doing a more active practice and you enjoy restorative poses, include one or two at the end of your practice. Select poses that you can hold for longer amounts of time so that you can relax completely and use appropriate propping to ensure your comfort.

For more information on both restorative and supported inverted poses described above, see "How to Practice Restorative Yoga and Supported Inverted Poses" later in this chapter on page 149.

CONSCIOUS RELAXATION. Guided relaxation, meditation, calming breath practices, and Relaxation Pose with a mental focus are practices that you can do on their own or include in an active practice. Although these are effective techniques to end your practice with, you can also use them to start a practice as a way to center yourself. Use the ones that work best for you and your particular circumstances (maybe you're on an airplane, for example), and make sure to use seated or reclined positions that you can hold for extended periods so you can relax completely. If necessary, use appropriate propping so you can practice comfortably. See "How to Practice Relaxation Pose" on page 144.

CALMING PRACTICE

This sequence is designed to quiet your nervous system and relax your body by combining supported inverted poses, including Standing Forward Bend, Bridge Pose, and Legs Up the Wall Pose, and to reduce your overall stress levels with restorative poses, including Reclined Twist and Child's Pose.

As you practice, make sure you're completely comfortable in all the poses, taking time to adjust your props if necessary. If you are uncomfortable with straight legs in the Seated Forward Bend, add a blanket roll under your knees. We recommend that you choose a mental focus, such as your breath or a mantra, to use with poses in which you're spending an extended amount of time.

For information on exhalation lengthening, see "Exhalation Lengthening" on page 176. For information about breath awareness, see "How to Practice Breath Awareness" on page 146.

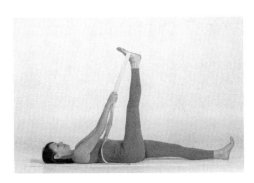

1. Reclined Leg Stretch, version 1, 1–2 minutes each side

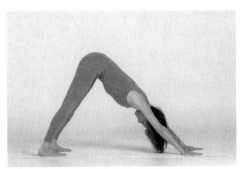

2. Downward-Facing Dog Pose, version 1, 2, or 3, 1–2 minutes

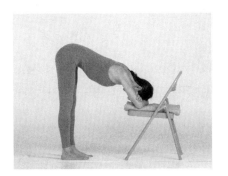

3. Standing Forward Bend, version 4, 1–2 minutes

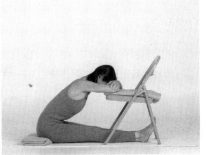

4. Seated Forward Bend, version 4, 2–3 minutes

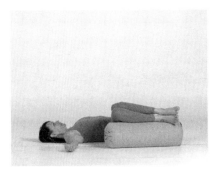

5. Reclined Twist, version 4, 2 minutes each side

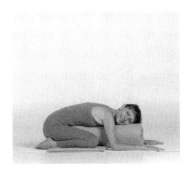

6. Child's Pose, version 4, 2–3 minutes

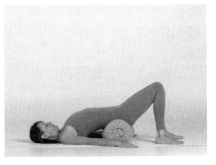

7. Bridge Pose, version 4, 2–3 minutes

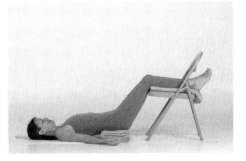

8. Legs Up the Wall Pose, version 4, exhalation lengthening, 3–5 minutes

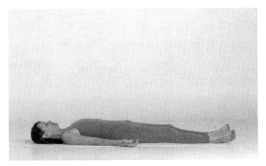

9. Relaxation Pose, any version, breath awareness, 5–10 minutes

HOW TO PRACTICE RELAXATION POSE

Relaxation Pose is often just an afterthought for many of us, especially in public classes where we quickly wrap up a practice by "lying down" for just a few minutes. But this pose can be very powerful. When you practice it with a mental focus, you can trigger the relaxation response. Relaxation Pose also allows you to relax your entire body in an anatomically neutral position, which provides deep physical rest. And as a form of reclined meditation, it can teach you about the way your mind works, just as seated meditation does.

Preparing to Practice

Although Relaxation Pose can be practiced on its own, we typically do it at the end of an asana practice. That's because it is often hard for us to lie still for a long period of time if we haven't exercised much. But keep in mind that what you should practice before Relaxation Pose depends on the time of day and what you have already been doing or not doing.

If you want to practice first thing in the morning or if you have had a sedentary day, you should prepare for Relaxation Pose with an active practice, which will tire you out and allow you to rest more comfortably. Strength-building sequences with challenging poses or long holds or agility practices with dynamic poses and flow sequences will be helpful at this time.

On the other hand, if you have had a strenuous day physically, either doing physical labor or standing on your feet all day, a practice focused on gentle stretching is a good way to release held tension from your body. For example, try sequences such as our Upper Body and Lower Body Flexibility sequences. If you are really exhausted, a restorative practice may be right for you.

Finally, if you are very stressed out, calming your nervous system is your priority; otherwise, it will definitely be hard to lie still. In this case, practicing supported inverted poses, such as Legs Up the Wall Pose, will help calm you down enough so that you can lie still. In general, before practicing, take some time to consider what feels right to you at that moment and follow your intuition.

Choosing a Version

Many people cannot be truly comfortable lying flat on the floor with no support. So the next step is to choose the right version of Relaxation Pose for your body and for the particular day and time. See page 256 for our four versions of Relaxation Pose.

If you can't get comfortable on your back or shouldn't lie on your back for some reason (for example, because you are pregnant), you can try a side-lying position instead. If you find that lying on your back causes anxiety, you can try a prone position (lying on your belly). If the room is cold, dress warmly, wear socks, and even cover yourself with a blanket.

To receive the full benefits of Relaxation Pose, you need to practice it with intention (rather than just collapsing onto the floor). To do this, commit to the following practices.

Aligning your body

Position your legs eight to ten inches apart, turn your arms out so your palms face up and your hands are six to eight inches from your body, with your head evenly between your shoulders and facing straight up toward the ceiling (not turning to one side). None of us are completely symmetrical, but you can adjust your body so it's as symmetrical as possible with your weight evenly distributed on both sides of your body. Now your alignment is close to what medical books call "anatomical neutral," the position your body naturally assumes when no muscles are being activated. When you are in this neutral position, you can begin to relax your body completely.

Remaining still

After aligning your body, make a commitment to stay still. When your body becomes motionless, external stimulation is reduced to a minimum, allowing your nervous system to calm down and your mind to quiet.

Using a mental focus

After you've aligned and quieted your body, turn your awareness inward. Typically the focus for your mind in Relaxation Pose is your breath, the gradual relaxation of specific parts of your body (sometimes called a body scan), or a peaceful image (for example, you might imagine your mind is the surface of a lake whose ripples are slowly subsiding). Rather than simply letting your thoughts wander as they would if you were lying on the grass in a park, intentionally keep your mind on your chosen focus. When you notice your attention wandering, gently return it to that focus.

Maintaining your awareness as you come out of the pose

If possible, stay in the pose for at least ten minutes. When you are ready to come out, open your eyes to passively receive the light of the room. Then let your body know you're ready to begin moving by gently wiggling just your fingers and toes or simply taking a couple of deep soft breaths. Next, bend your knees and place the soles of your feet on the ground and then slowly turn over onto your right side and rest there for a couple of breaths. Then slowly use your hands to push yourself up to a seated position, allowing your head to release downward until you are completely upright. Finally, when you are upright, slowly lift your head.

HOW TO PRACTICE BREATH AWARENESS

Simple breath awareness is a practice of observing your breath without changing it. With formal breath practices (pranayama), you intentionally change your breathing patterns by making your inhalations and/or exhalations longer, holding your breath, or breathing in a special fashion (such as humming, alternating nostrils, and so on), which typically has a stronger effect on your nervous system. With simple breath awareness, you just watch your natural breathing patterns, which is very effective and completely safe.

Breath awareness can be used in two different ways: as a meditation technique or as a stress management technique. Ten to twenty minutes of simple breath awareness will trigger the relaxation response, quieting both your nervous system and your mind. Even a few minutes of practice can help center you or head off a spike in your stress levels. Nina Rook, who in the past suffered from anxiety, says, "The most powerful and immediate antidote for anxiety is simply breathing—when I focus on my breath, that focus disrupts and displaces the anxiety loops."[3]

Whether you are practicing breath awareness for stress management or as a form of meditation, the way you practice will depend on your location and position. This section will help you choose the best location and positions for stress management (see chapter 10 for the best location, position, and timing for meditation). It concludes with information about choosing a focus, which applies to both stress management and meditation.

Choosing Your Location

You don't need a special location to practice breath awareness. As long as there is a quiet spot for you to sit—whether on the floor, out in nature, or on a chair—you can practice. You can also practice breath awareness while you are doing your favorite restorative pose or even while you are in bed as a way to soothe yourself to sleep (or back to sleep).

When you're traveling or are stuck somewhere busy and noisy, such as at your office or on a train or an airplane, you can practice there, too.

It's more challenging when there are distractions or you are in a public place, but it is still an effective way to calm yourself in the middle of a hectic day.

Choosing Your Position

The position you choose will depend on your location. You have the most options in a house, where you can practice in a yoga sitting pose, a restorative pose, sitting on a chair, or lying on your bed. Obviously, if you are at work or some other public place, you may have to limit yourself to sitting on a chair.

Sitting

Our recommended positions for seated breath awareness are Easy Sitting Pose and Hero Pose. We have provided comfortable variations of these poses using props, which should allow you stay in the pose for longer periods of time. (See part 2 for more options.)

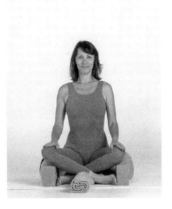
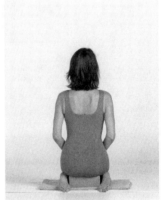

If you can't get comfortable on the floor or if the current setting doesn't allow it, sitting on a chair is always an option. But rather than leaning against the back of the chair and slumping, sit on the front edge of the chair with your feet flat on the floor (if you are short, you might need to put a prop under them, or if your legs are long, you might need to put some padding on the chair seat), with your spine resting in its natural curves, and your head in line with your spine. Obviously someone with physical disabilities can practice breath awareness in whatever position they are able to take, in whatever chair they happen to be.

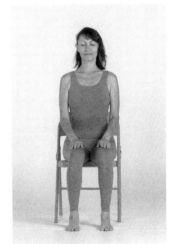

Restorative Poses

You can practice breath awareness in any restorative yoga pose that you find comfortable, as well as in gentle supported inverted poses, such as Legs Up the Wall Pose. We especially recommend Reclined Cobbler's Pose and Relaxation Pose with support.

If you're someone who tends to be anxious and lying on your back makes you feel vulnerable or if you can't lie on your back for some reason, Supported Child's Pose is a good alternative. This will allow you to bring awareness to your breath in your back body, which can be more relaxing for anxious people.

In Bed

You can practice breath awareness under the covers in your bed, in your customary sleeping position. This is a good way to improve your sleep because you will fall asleep in a more relaxed state or to get back to sleep if you wake in the middle of the night. Depending on what's most comfortable for you, practice either on your back with your head supported by a pillow or lying on your side with a pillow between your legs.

Standing

If you just want to center yourself—or help head off a spike in stress—you can practice breath awareness anytime and anywhere in Mountain Pose. Because standing still for ten to twenty minutes is very challenging, this position is best for a short, "quick fix" session of breath awareness.

Choosing Your Focus

What does it mean to bring your awareness to your breath? There are actually many options to explore either the quality of your breath or the way your breath moves in your body. Try out the various techniques listed below to find one that engages your attention but doesn't make you feel anxious about your breathing. As you observe your breath, consciously refrain from changing it. You may notice, however, that as time goes on, your breathing pattern may change on its own because you are relaxing more and more.

For all techniques, be sure to maintain a nonjudgmental attitude about your ability to concentrate. If you want to trigger the relaxation response, continue practicing for ten to twenty minutes. If you just want to center yourself, a shorter period of time—even just one minute—will be effective.

Feeling your body respond to your breath

For beginners, probably the easiest way to observe the breath is to watch the dramatic way your body moves as your lungs expand and shrink. As you inhale and exhale, you can feel your belly rise and fall, your chest expand and shrink back, or your ribs move out to the sides and back again. In positions where you are lying on your side or are prone (Child's Pose), an interesting option is to feel your back rise and fall with your breath. This may be a soothing choice for those who tend to be anxious.

Sound

If it is quiet enough, you can focus on listening to the internal sounds you make as you breathe in and out.

Feeling your breath itself

The best way to "feel" your actual breath is to bring awareness to the sensations in your nostrils, sensing the air flowing in and out of them. You can also notice the quality of the breath moving in and out of your lungs. Is it smooth or rough? Relaxed or forced? Is your exhalation or inhalation longer than the other, or are they the same duration?

RESTORATIVE YOGA AND SUPPORTED INVERTED POSES

This section provides background information about restorative yoga and supported inverted poses, tips about practicing, and sequences that you can practice to experience their effects.

Restorative Yoga

Restorative yoga was specially created to provide deep rest and relaxation. When practicing, you use props to support yourself in classic yoga poses, including forward bends, backbends, side stretches, twists, and inversions. For example, in the restorative version of Child's Pose, rather than folding forward all the way onto the floor, you use a bolster or stack of folded blankets to support your entire front body.

The props you use in restorative yoga not only make the pose more comfortable but also take the effort out of the pose. Rather than you using your muscles to hold yourself in the shape of a pose, the props hold you in the pose so you can simply let your muscles relax. You can then turn your attention inward, focusing on your breath, physical sensations, or any other object of meditation, which triggers the relaxation response.

Because you typically stay in a restorative yoga pose for longer periods of time than in an active one, the emotional effect can be stronger. For example, the forward bend of Child's Pose is normally quieting, but the restorative version is even more so. Active backbends can be stimulating and uplifting, and while the restorative versions are not stimulating, if you are set up properly, a restorative backbend can be uplifting, providing an antidepressant effect. (See "Asanas and Your Emotions" on page 182 for information on the emotional effects of poses.)

Finally, in a restorative pose, you still receive many of the benefits of the pose itself. For example, in a restorative backbend, you are opening your chest and stretching many of the muscles that become tight after driving long distances or sitting hunched forward at a desk all day. Passively stretching your muscles as you unwind increases your feeling of relaxation, as some of the stress you have been holding in your body is gently released. Because you are completely comfortable and relaxed, you can stay in the pose for much longer, so restorative poses are actually a good way to work on flexibility as well as relaxation.

Restorative yoga is perfect for those days when you feel depleted, sick, stressed out, low on energy, or are just in the mood for a soothing practice. For people who can't practice inversions for stress reduction, restorative yoga poses are an excellent alternative. For example, Reclined Cobbler's Pose with props is the perfect choice for a ten- to twenty-minute stress reduction practice. But if you're feeling hyper from stress or anxiety, you may find it difficult to lie down in a restorative pose. In this case, we recommend doing either an active yoga practice or some other form of exercise before doing the restorative pose.

TIMING. If you are new to yoga, start by holding the poses for one to two minutes and gradually lengthen your time. For experienced practitioners, use your present practice times as a starting point and, if it works for you, gradually increase your time in the poses.

You may need to experiment a bit to find your maximum timing for these poses. For some restorative poses, such as Supported Child's Pose or version 4 of Reclined Twist, you'll find that four to five minutes is long enough and that you become uncomfortable after that. However, for Reclined Cobbler's Pose and the supported versions of Relaxation Pose, which are typically very comfortable for longer holds, we recommend that you work toward ten-minute holds to trigger the relaxation response. If you are still completely comfortable, feel free to stay in the poses even longer. Some experienced yoga practitioners will stay in Reclined Cobbler's Pose for forty-five minutes! Just don't allow yourself to fall asleep in the pose, as you can overstretch.

RESTORATIVE YOGA PRACTICE

This sequence focuses on supported poses that relax your body while they quiet your nervous system. The restorative poses in this sequence gently release tension in the front and back of your body, especially the lower back, hamstrings, abdomen, and chest. In addition to using this sequence for general relaxation, you can also use it for quieting your digestive system and supporting your immune system. As you practice, focus on your breath and on deepening the feelings of physical relaxation throughout your body.

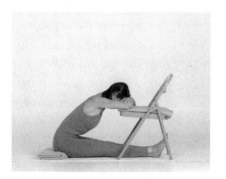

1. Supported Backbend, version 1 or 3, 2–4 minutes

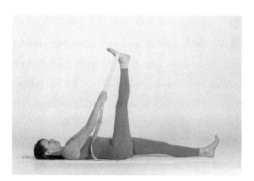

2. Reclined Leg Stretch, version 1, 1–2 minutes

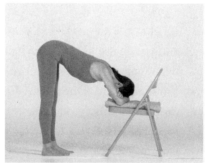

3. Standing Forward Bend, version 4, 1–3 minutes

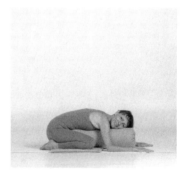

4. Child's Pose, version 4, 1–3 minutes

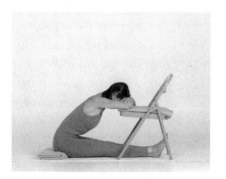

5. Seated Forward Bend, version 4, 1–3 minutes

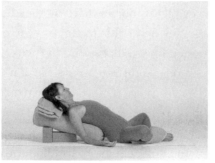

6. Reclined Cobbler's Pose, version 2, 3, or 4, 5–20 minutes

Supported Inverted Poses

The supported inverted poses are a special class of restorative poses. In an inverted pose, your heart is higher than your head, the opposite of its position when you are sitting or standing. These poses tend to be naturally calming because they cause the blood from the parts of your body that are above your head to flow toward your head, which will automatically trigger the relaxation response if you stay in the pose for a while. As long as you are warm, quiet, and comfortable in the inverted pose, all you have to do is let the pose work its magic. Some find that the relaxation achieved with these poses is more refreshing than that from other types of restorative poses, although not everyone agrees!

The supported versions of the inverted poses are almost always more relaxing than the versions in which you must support yourself. For example, Standing Forward Bend with your head and arms resting on a chair is far more calming for most people than the classic version. So for restorative practices or for relaxation at the end of an active sequence, we recommend practicing the supported versions of inverted poses. Although we don't have any full inversions in our book (the classics are Headstand and Shoulderstand), we do include partial and gentle inversions.

PARTIAL INVERSIONS. Partial inversions are poses where your heart and pelvis are above your head, but your feet are below your heart. We have included three supported partial inversions in this book: Standing Forward Bend, Downward-Facing Dog Pose, and Bridge Pose. Although they are soothing on their own, they are also good warm-ups for gentle inversions (see the following section) because they stretch the backs of your legs and open your shoulders and hips. They also allow you to gradually become accustomed to being partly upside down.

GENTLE INVERSIONS. Gentle inversions are poses where your heart is only slightly higher than your head. Because these poses are more gradual, they are accessible to almost everyone. We have included two gentle supported inverted poses in this book: Legs Up the Wall Pose (four different versions) and Bridge Pose, version 4. The advantage of these poses is that they are very comfortable for most people, and you can stay in them for quite a while. Some people find that after seven to eight minutes, they can actually feel the relaxation response kick in.

You don't need to warm up for these poses, but you may be more comfortable if you do. Although we typically include them near the end of a sequence, you can practice them at the beginning of a sequence or even just on their own as a one-pose practice.

TIMING. If you are new to yoga, start out by holding the supported inverted poses for thirty seconds and gradually work your way to longer holds of five to ten minutes, as long as the pose is comfortable. If you are an experienced practitioner you can use your present practice times as a starting point and, if it works for you, gradually increase your time in the poses. Ultimately, you should aim to hold a pose long enough to trigger the relaxation response—about ten minutes. If you are still comfortable after that, feel free to stay in the pose even longer. Some experienced yoga practitioners will stay in Legs Up the Wall Pose for twenty minutes!

SUPPORTED INVERSIONS PRACTICE

This sequence is designed to maximize the relaxing effects of supported inverted poses by combining them all into a single practice. The more time you spend in these poses, the deeper your feeling of relaxation will be. The first two poses stretch your shoulders and legs to make the supported inversions more comfortable for you. You then ease one pose at a time from a partial inversion to an almost full inversion, becoming more and more quiet as you go. As you practice, focus on the quality of your breath, especially in the final Legs Up the Wall Pose.

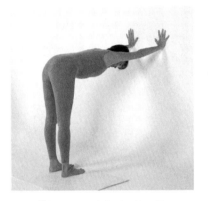

1. Half Downward-Facing Dog Pose, any version, 1 minute

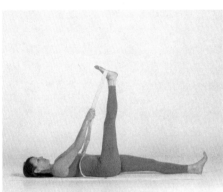

2. Reclined Leg Stretch, version 1, 1–2 minutes

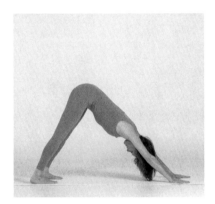

3. Downward-Facing Dog Pose, any version, 1–2 minutes

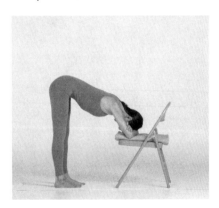

4. Standing Forward Bend, version 4, 1–3 minutes

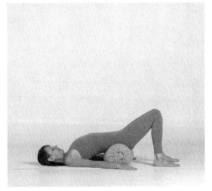

5. Bridge Pose, version 4, 3–5 minutes

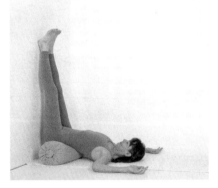

6. Legs Up the Wall Pose, any version, 5–20 minutes

YOGA FOR BETTER SLEEP

Even though spending time awake in the rest-and-digest state is vital for your physical, mental, and emotional health, so is getting enough sleep! Fortunately, the two activities are complementary, as using conscious relaxation techniques can actually help improve the quality of your sleep. That's why yoga can be especially beneficial for people with sleep problems. We know that when you're having problems sleeping, taking time to relax rather than just trying to get more sleep seems counterintuitive. But, trust us, because insomnia is often a result of chronic stress, taking the time to practice yoga for better sleep will improve your nights as well as your days. Here are some tips to help you get started:

1. Reduce your overall stress levels—Start by using the techniques we recommended in this chapter for reducing chronic stress on a regular basis. This can help prevent the busy mind and overstimulated nervous system that keep you awake at night.

2. Plan your day—What you do in the hours before you go to bed can affect your state when you get into bed. So schedule your stimulating activities, including aerobic exercise and strong yoga practices, such as standing poses, flow practices, and backbends, for earlier in the day. (Of course, you don't want to be watching an action film in the late evening, either.) Start to wind down before bed with calming practices, such as restorative yoga or meditation, so you're in a relaxed state when you get into bed.

3. Get comfortable—Physical pain or discomfort can keep you awake, so think about your sleeping position the same way you would about a yoga pose. Use "props" in bed, such as extra pillows, towels, and so on, to help get more comfortable. If you are having back problems, you can exacerbate them by sleeping on your belly and overarching your lower back. You could try placing a folded blanket or towel under your lower abdomen to see if that helps, or, even better, sleep on your back instead with a pillow under your knees. If you're having neck problems, sleep on your side or back, rather than on your belly. If you try sleeping on your side and find that your knees press together uncomfortably, place a pillow between your knees. If nocturnal leg cramps are keeping you awake, stretch your legs before bed.

4. Practice yoga in bed—Sometimes just getting into bed, even if you've been relaxing beforehand, can trigger worries about your life or fear about falling asleep. Instead of letting your mind race,

try your favorite relaxation practice while you're falling asleep (in this case, it's okay if you fall asleep while you're relaxing). You could practice guided relaxation (by listening to an audio recording or just talking yourself through it) or even do a restorative yoga pose, such as Supported Child's Pose, with a mental focus to calm yourself down.

5. Work with your breath—One of the easiest things you can do to calm yourself before you fall asleep or if you wake up in the middle of the night is to work with your breath. This moves your mind away from your worries onto a neutral subject and triggers the relaxation response, which will help you fall asleep more quickly and sleep more deeply. You can either practice simple breath awareness or gently lengthen your exhalation (see "Exhalation Lengthening" on page 176). If you have trouble breathing because you have a cold or allergies, try working with a mantra (a phrase you repeat to yourself) instead.

YOGA FOR HEALTHY EATING

Chronic stress can not only cause digestive problems, but it can also trigger the release of cortisol, which can cause overeating and weight gain by stimulating your appetite. Using your yoga practice to reduce your stress and cortisol levels is one of the most important things you can do to move toward healthy eating. Debbie Cabusas says that soon after she started regularly practicing calming and balancing pranayama, she noticed her sugar cravings were pretty much gone. As she continued to practice regularly, almost all her cravings disappeared, and she began to lose weight. For healthy eating, practice any stress management techniques that are effective in reducing your chronic stress. For those who want further help, here are a couple of other tips.

Mindfulness

Many poor eating habits are just that—habits! Practicing yoga poses mindfully and meditating as described in chapter 10 will help you tune in to your body instead of ignoring it. Elizabeth D., who lost fifty pounds and has been able to keep it off, says that her regular meditation practice manages her stress and helps her be more aware of how she's feeling, leading to better eating choices. She says, "Most of the time, when I'm hungry, I'm actually dehydrated or have low potassium. I'll have a glass of water and a banana, and I'm fine."

As you tune in to your body, you may realize that foods you are currently eating are compromising your health or notice poor eating habits, such as eating beyond satiety. Cultivating mindfulness can teach you to recognize:

- Which foods are good for you and which are not (whether that means junk food or food to which you are allergic or intolerant)
- When you are full and don't need to eat more
- When you are thirsty instead of hungry
- When you are eating for stress, not for hunger

Mindfulness will also help you start to recognize habitual thoughts that are getting in the way of healthy eating. You can then work on changing your perspective (see "Practice" in chapter 11).

Willpower

Once you've identified your habits or have decided to eliminate or cut back on certain foods, it takes willpower to change! According to Dr. Kelly McGonigal, being in a state of stress can increase impulsive behavior and decrease willpower. Practicing stress management as we described above will help with your willpower. However, you can also use a meditation practice to intentionally strengthen your willpower. Meditation teaches you to return to your object of focus and tune out distractions, or temptations. Research has also demonstrated that as little as three hours of accumulated meditation can improve willpower. Dr. McGonigal says:

> Neuroscientists have discovered that when you ask the brain to meditate, it gets better not just at meditating, but at a wide range of self-control skills, including attention, focus, stress management, impulse control, and self-awareness. People who meditate regularly aren't just better at these things. Over time, their brains become finely tuned willpower machines. Regular meditators have more gray matter in the prefrontal cortex, as well as regions of the brain that support self-awareness.[4]

Cultivating Equanimity

Six months after Hurricane Katrina, Mary Ann Avallone-O'Gorman was still "ankle deep in mud and devastation." Her house was gutted, her marriage was crumbling, and her daily life was a world of "bayou sludge, dead animals, rotten food, destroyed photographs." She was dealing with it all by pretending she had "superpowers," spending long hours doing intense physical labor, eating take-out food, and drinking a lot of wine. Then, on impulse one evening she took a gentle basic yoga class.

At the end of the class when she lay down in the final pose, Savasana, she noticed that she felt "cocooned" and safe for the first time in months. As her teacher talked the class through the pose, she began sobbing and could not stop even as she left the class and drove home. Then later that night, she had an epiphany: "My successful attempts at strongarming through all adversity—through natural disasters and relationship disasters—painted me into a corner. The only way out was to soften into ease and grace."

Now, ten years later, Mary Ann is a yoga teacher as well as a dedicated practitioner. She tells her students:

> You bring your whole life to the mat. Your wisdom. Your strength. Your failures. Your attitude about all these things. Use what serves

Yoga, of course, is so much more than postures, and its real power lies in the domain of mind training and self-transformation.

—Georg Feuerstein, *The Deeper Dimension of Yoga*

you. Observe what does not. Place it gently to the side. That act, in itself, is a yogic practice. Recognize all the traits you bring to all that you do. Allow your yoga practice to be exactly that: a practice of and for your whole life.[1]

The Bhagavad Gita defines *yoga* as "equanimity" and tells us that equanimity allows us to face difficulty with a "steady and quiet" mind:

> He who hates not light, nor busy activity, nor even darkness, when they are near, neither longs for them when they are far.
>
> Who unperturbed by changing conditions sits apart and watches and says "the powers of nature go round," and remains firm and shakes not.
>
> Who dwells in his inner self, and is the same in pleasure and pain; to whom gold or stones or earth are one, and what is pleasing or displeasing leave him in peace; who is beyond both praise and blame, and whose mind is steady and quiet.[2]

Although many of us will never have to deal with a disaster of the magnitude of Hurricane Katrina, we all have to deal with adversity throughout our lives. So whatever our age, it will benefit us all tremendously to learn to face difficulty with as much equanimity as possible.

While we do believe that yoga has many answers for helping us age gracefully, we hope you realize by now that we are also realists about both the "aging" and "yoga" parts of our mission. We know that even if we can extend our health spans through healthy practices, almost all of us will have to go through poor health at some point. We know that even if we can prolong our independence into old age, many of us will eventually have to face the loss of that, however briefly. We know that even if we are ourselves blessed with long and healthy lives, we'll all have to deal with losing people we love. And then there are the little day-to-day problems! That is why we feel that cultivating equanimity through wisdom and practice is the most important pillar of healthy aging.

This chapter discusses how cultivating equanimity can help you work with and accept difficulty and become more content with what you have and don't have. According to The Yoga Sutras, this leads to happiness:

> From contentment and benevolence of consciousness comes supreme happiness.[3]

Yoga has evolved quite dramatically since that text was written. New practices, such as restorative yoga and supported inverted poses, and new ways of doing old practices, such as guided forms of Relaxation Pose, are now part of the yoga lexicon. All of these techniques work in different ways and have somewhat different effects, so let's begin with a quick overview of the ones we recommend:

- Stress management—As conscious relaxation practices calm your nervous system, they also quiet your mind and help reduce feelings of stress, anxiety, depression, and anger. If chronic stress is causing you to lose your cool, either mentally or emotionally, practicing yoga for stress management is a good place in your journey to cultivate equanimity. Then, whenever you're ready, you can add in any of our equanimity practices.

- Meditation—Meditation is an effective way to trigger the relaxation response, calming your nervous system and quieting your mind, but more importantly it allows you to study your mind and gain more control over it. This chapter provides information about the many benefits of meditation and detailed instructions for how to practice it.

- Mindful asanas—Practicing yoga mindfully as a form of moving meditation is a very powerful tool for improving your mental and emotional health as well as your physical health. When you systematically pay attention to your body, you will learn what it is telling you—if you are stressed, anxious, angry, and so on—and become better able to take appropriate steps to bring yourself back into balance. Practicing this way also helps you cultivate your inner witness, which you can use to train your nervous system to react more calmly to stressful situations. This chapter provides instructions for mindfully practicing yoga.

- Pranayama—You can use specific practices to stimulate, calm, or balance yourself, allowing you to manage your energy levels and moods. This chapter explains why breath practices have such a powerful effect and provides detailed instructions on the breath practices that we recommend.

- Asanas for emotional balance—Because different types of poses have different effects on your emotions and energy levels, you can use your asana practice to stimulate yourself when you're feeling lethargic, to calm yourself when you're feeling hyper, and to uplift yourself when you're feeling down. This chapter provides general guidelines on how to use the different types of poses to influence your emotions.

- Yoga philosophy—Studying yoga philosophy provides you with an alternative way of thinking about your life, enabling you to be more content with what you have and what you don't have and to become more comfortable with change. The classic yoga texts also provide useful insights into the nature of the mind, which you can use to help change your mental habits and behavioral patterns. (See chapter 11 for more information.)

This chapter provides information on cultivating equanimity with meditation, mindful asana practice, pranayama, and poses for emotional balance. It concludes with some general advice on self-regulation.

Before she practiced yoga, Nina Rook was stressed out and anxious due to a demanding career, daily life as a working mother, and a marriage that was coming to an end. Now she says:

> By maintaining a practice that brings me into the present and into acute awareness of my body and my mind, I believe that I dampen anxiety about the future. I even experience some degree of contentment (santosha), the *niyama* that "brings unsurpassed joy." But this is not a "what will be, will be" acceptance. It hums with energy: being aware of the good as well as the bad in any situation, focusing on my thought patterns, taking steps to maintain the physical health, which keeps more options possible.[4]

MEDITATION

He who restrains well the mind, [which is] far-going, wide-roaming, of the essence of desire and doubt—he is happy here [on Earth] and in the hereafter.

—Georg Feuerstein, translator, "Moksha-Dharma," *The Yoga Tradition*

Anyone who studies even a little history of yoga will soon learn that the aim of the original yogis was to quiet the mind. Although in chapter 9 we recommended meditation as a technique for triggering the relaxation response, meditation has the power to do so much more than just calm you down.

Because the mind is typically busy with thoughts, many of which disturb your equanimity—regrets about the past, worries about the future, and dissatisfaction with the present—using meditation to quiet your mind allows you to experience feelings of peace and contentment. Meditation also fosters a feeling of compassion, which improves your relationships with others, and a feeling of gratitude, which allows you to be more content with what you have and what you don't have. In addition, the process of meditating allows you to observe your habitual thought patterns and emotional responses, which is the first step in changing them to more positive ones. This section discusses the four different ways you can use meditation for cultivating equanimity along with specific instructions on how to meditate.

Quieting the Mind

In sutra 1.2 of The Yoga Sutras, Patanjali wrote:

> Yoga is the stilling of the changing states of the mind.[5]

Stilling the changing "states of mind"—also translated as the "whirls of consciousness"—means quieting the thoughts that cycle over and over in your mind. While not all our thoughts disturb our equanimity, when we are worried, anxious, sad, depressed, or even overly excited, we can be tormented by thoughts and emotions that whirl uncontrollably through us. In classical yoga, quieting the mind is recommended as the antidote to the *kleshas*, our reactions to life that disturb our equanimity and are the source of our suffering. (See chapter 11 for a discussion of this sutra and what quieting the mind means in classical yoga.)

The simple act of regular meditation quiets your mind, but you may find that certain techniques work more effectively for you than others, depending on your particular personality or even just your current circumstances. You may wish to experiment with several different techniques, perhaps even keeping a record of your state of mind before and after practice for several days in a row.

Self-Study with Meditation

By using your witness mind as you meditate, you can engage in self-study (*svadhyaya*) to learn about habitual thought patterns and emotional responses that you might not even be aware of.

The witness mind is that part of our minds that allows us to observe ourselves in action while we are acting. The Sanskrit word for witness is *sakshi*, and it refers to the "pure awareness" that witnesses the world without being affected by it or involved with it. The word *sakshi* is a combination of two other words: *sa* and *aksha*. *Sa* means "with" and *aksha* means "eyes." So sakshi is awareness that can observe "with its own eyes." A second meaning of *aksha* is "the center of a wheel." Because the center of a wheel remains still as the wheel turns, sakshi, the witness mind, is awareness that remains steady while events turn around it.

In meditation, your witness mind observes when your attention has wandered from the object of your meditation—and to what. Rather than floating down the stream of your thoughts, you sit on the shore and impartially observe from a distance. As you observe with detachment what's happening within you—your sensations, thoughts, and emotions—you start to recognize patterns that you may later decide to change. Observing your habits can help you change your general patterns of reactivity, especially the way you react to stress. All of this will help you cultivate equanimity in your daily life.

You can also use your witness mind during your asana practice. To do this, as you practice, summon your witness mind to observe your reactions to the poses you're practicing and to notice when your mind is wandering away from your presence in the yoga room. Eventually you can use your witness mind in the same way during any activity.

Compassion

Sutra 1.33 of The Yoga Sutras says the following:

> By cultivating an attitude of friendship toward those who are happy, compassion toward those in distress, joy toward those who are virtuous, and equanimity toward those who are nonvirtuous, lucidity arises in the mind.[6]

In addition to quieting your mind and teaching you about your thought patterns, meditation provides interpersonal benefits. Studies have shown that the practice of meditation increases compassion, and becoming more compassionate clearly fosters better relationships with people in your life as well as strangers who are suffering. Scientists who have studied this phenomenon speculate that there are two possible explanations for this. The first is that because meditation improves your ability to pay attention, it might improve your ability to notice what's going on with someone else (as opposed to being lost in your own thoughts). Another explanation is that meditation helps us to experience the interconnectedness of all beings.

Interestingly, one study showed that when people meditated on "non-referential" compassion, the regions of their brains responsible for planned action were activated, as if they were preparing to aid people in distress. So you may find yourself with an urge to help others—always a good thing, both for them and you.

A regular meditation practice of any kind will foster compassion, but if you wish to work on this intentionally, you could do the following:

- Choose a person for whom you wish to cultivate compassion, and before meditating set the intention that your practice will be dedicated to them. Then check in after you finish by holding that person in your mind again.
- Use the word *compassion* as a mantra.
- Practice the loving-kindness meditation, a structured meditation

designed to help you open your heart and cultivate compassion toward people close to you as well as strangers. (You can find instructions on how to practice the loving-kindness meditation in many books on meditation.)
- Practice any other formal meditation designed to foster compassion.

Gratitude

Meditating on gratitude can have a profound effect on your mood and state of mind. In fact, scientists have actually identified biochemical explanations for this. They've discovered that feelings of gratitude activate the part of the brain that produces dopamine, a messenger molecule that stimulates your brain's reward and pleasure center. Feeling gratitude toward others also stimulates your social dopamine circuits, making your social interactions more pleasurable. Even thinking of things to be grateful for boosts your serotonin levels, increasing your happiness.

To cultivate gratitude in your meditation practice, you can use the following techniques:

- Use the word *gratitude* as a mantra.
- Choose one thing for which you are grateful and use it as the object of your meditation, either as a mantra or as an image.
- Set the intention that as you meditate you will notice things you are grateful for as they naturally arise in your mind.
- Practice any formal meditation practice designed to cultivate gratitude.

Of course, when you are being harassed by negative thoughts, it often isn't easy to find and focus on things you are grateful for, but apparently the effort of remembering to look for gratitude alone provides the benefits. Just like strengthening a muscle, practicing gratitude regularly makes you stronger at being grateful over time, so you'll be improving your gratitude practice as you age!

HOW TO MEDITATE

This section describes the options you have when you want to meditate. Because the environment in which you'll be meditating will influence the position you take and the object of meditation you choose, we'll start by discussing settings. We'll then address position, mental focus, timing, and meditation itself.

Choose Your Setting

You probably have an image of the perfect quiet, warm, clean environment in which you should meditate, but real life doesn't always present that. If you can't set up a separate space because you live in a small apartment or a crowded family house, you shouldn't let that stop you from practicing. As long as there is room for you to sit—whether on the floor or even on a chair—you can meditate.

If you can set up a separate quiet space for your meditating practice, by all means do so, but if not, just do the best you can. When you're traveling or are stuck somewhere busy and noisy, such as at an airport or even on an airplane, go ahead and practice there, too. It's more challenging to practice when there are distractions or you are in a public place, but it is still practicing, and in fact it's probably a more realistic way of learning to quiet your mind. As our colleague Ram Rao said:

> The goal of meditation is to be at ease, relaxed, and at peace with our surroundings. It is important to not resist the disturbing/distracting influence that comes in the way of your meditation practice. So do not try to ignore the influence or to block it out, for if you try, you will only meet with stiffer resistance, ending in frustration. Instead, simply let it be (*thathaasthu*, in Sanskrit) and continue with your meditation. Everything is a part of meditation, all the influences including the noise, the thoughts, the emotions, and the resistance from the mind. Treat everything that arises in meditation the same way—let it be and just be there![7]

Choose Your Position

Typically people meditate in a seated position on the floor. This is simply because an upright, unsupported position allows you to quiet your mind without falling asleep. For those who can't sit for long periods without major discomfort, reclining is also an option if you're in the right environment. For short meditations, you can meditate standing up. Obviously your environment affects your position choice, as sometimes your options are limited.

SEATED POSITIONS. Our recommended positions for seated meditation are Easy Sitting Pose and Hero Pose (although a few people are comfortable enough to meditate in Half Lotus or even Full Lotus). For both of those poses, we have provided a comfortable variation using props, which should allow you stay in the pose for longer periods of time (see part 2 for more options).

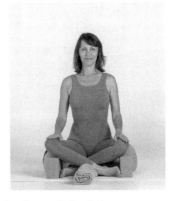
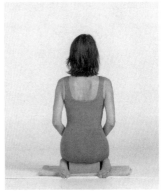

For people who just can't get comfortable on the floor—or who can't get down to and up from the floor—sitting on a chair is always an option. Instead of leaning against the back of the chair, sit on the front edge of the chair with your feet flat on the floor (put a prop under them if you're short or put some padding on the chair seat if your legs are long), with your spine resting in its natural curves, and your head in line with your spine. Someone with physical disabilities can meditate in whatever position they are able to take, in whatever chair they happen to be.

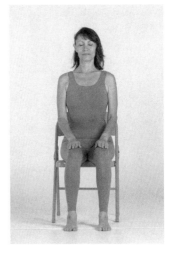

RECLINING POSITIONS. If you really can't get comfortable sitting down (or maybe you sit down all day for your work and just can't take it any longer), try a supine position. Because you want to avoid falling asleep, we feel that the best reclining position for meditation would be a supported form of Relaxation Pose where your head and heart are higher than your legs (as opposed to being flat on the floor or having your legs higher than your heart). So try lying down with your chest and head (but not your buttocks) on a bolster or on two blankets folded into long, thin rectangles. This will keep you a tiny bit stimulated and might help prevent you from falling asleep. But, as always, make sure the position is comfortable for you.

If you are someone who doesn't fall asleep during the day, you could try meditating in any reclined or even inverted position, such as Legs Up the Wall Pose, that you find comfortable, though these may only work for shorter meditations.

STANDING POSITIONS. Nina was recently surprised to see ancient statues of yogis meditating in Mountain Pose. It makes sense, if you think about it. After all, Buddhists meditate while walking or standing, so standing up to meditate is also an option if you have nowhere to sit or would just like to try something different. It is probably difficult to stand still for long periods of time, so for us normal mortals this position would only be effective for a short meditation.

Choose Your Focus

Different yogic traditions have different focuses and techniques for meditation. If you are already practicing meditation or following a certain tradition, you can simply continue using whatever technique you've been taught. However, if you are new to meditation or want to change things up, here are some suggestions.

BREATH. The breath is often recommended as a focus for beginners because it is always accessible and has no religious associations. You can focus on the sound of your breath, the sensations of your breath moving in and out of your nostrils, or the way your inhalations and exhalations affect your body, such as the rise and fall of your belly or the movement of your breastbone. But meditating on your breath doesn't work for everyone, and if you're ill or in pain, it may be better for you to take your mind off your body.

MANTRAS. Although there are traditional Sanskrit mantras used for meditation, you can use any word or phrase in any language that has a positive meaning for you. For example, Baxter uses the word *om* as well as his grandmother's name, Genevieve.

IMAGES. There are two ways to use an image as your focus. First, you can keep your eyes open and focus on an actual image before you, such as a candle flame or a piece of artwork. You can also meditate on an image you picture in your mind, such as a person or a natural setting that has meaning to you.

LENGTH OF TIME. If you're just starting a meditation practice, don't get caught up in how long to do it. The important thing is to start a new habit. As with all yoga practices, a little bit every day will bring greater benefits than longer sessions done intermittently. We recommend keeping it short and simple—just five or ten minutes at first. Set a timer so you don't have to worry about how long you've been meditating. As your habit becomes more established, you can gradually work up to twenty minutes a day or longer.

BASIC MEDITATION

After you have chosen your location, position, and mental focus, and have set your timer, simply follow these steps:

1. Commit to remaining still.
2. Focus on your chosen object of meditation—When you realize your mind is wandering (and it will wander), notice the thoughts you are

having and then, without judgment, gently guide your focus back to the object.

3. Stop when your timer goes off—After your practice session, refrain from judging how well it went. Instead, simply continue with your day.

If this practice is difficult for you, try not to get discouraged. You'll be learning about yourself no matter what. Dr. Herbert Benson's studies of the relaxation response, which he performed on people practicing mantra meditation, showed that even when practitioners didn't feel that they were doing a "good job" of meditating, they still gained the physiological benefits of lower blood pressure, slower heart rate, fewer stress hormones, and so on.

HOW TO PRACTICE YOGA POSES MINDFULLY

Practicing yoga poses mindfully keeps you in the present moment, allowing you to let go of regrets about the past, worries about the future, and judgments about the here and now. In general this is a good way to reduce your stress levels. But practicing poses mindfully is also a very powerful tool for improving your mental and emotional health as well as your physical health. Paying close attention to your body allows you to hear what it is telling you. Are you comfortable or are you uncomfortable, experiencing unusual physical symptoms, or even in pain? Are you content or are you irritated, stressed, or anxious? These messages will help you take the appropriate steps to bring yourself back into balance.

Many of us live in automatic-pilot mode, stuck in our heads with little awareness of what's going on with our bodies. If you are barely in touch with your body and unaware of how it is feeling most of the time, you won't realize how your environment, your interactions toward other people, and your own thoughts and feelings are affecting you. By systematically paying attention to your body in the yoga room, you will train yourself to be more tuned in to your body in general. You can use the appropriate yoga practices and techniques to respond.

Nina, for example, learned to recognize certain physical symptoms—a burning feeling in her chest and mild nausea—that tell her when she's overstressed. Now whenever she experiences those sensations, she knows it's time to scale back temporarily on stressful activities and focus instead on the yoga poses and breath practices that calm her down.

We recommend the following ways to practice yoga asanas mindfully:

A purposeful, regular yoga practice offered in a safe space with positive intention will shift any human being from a state of rigidity to flexibility, from overstressed, hyperstimulated, and hyperaroused toward increased feelings of stability and equanimity. This is because each time we practice physical postures we are invited to breathe intentionally and to turn our awareness toward sensations that arise in the body and observe thoughts that flow through the mind.

—C. J. Keller, Veteran's Yoga Project Ambassador, USMC

Practice at home. Practicing on your own, without the distraction of other people in the room or the teacher telling you what to do, forces you to pay more attention to your own experience of being in the poses.

Focus. If you are practicing at home, pick a single physical sensation to follow throughout your entire practice, whether it is the quality of your breath in every single pose, the even distribution of weight on your feet—the balls as well as the heels—in every pose, or even something more arcane. If you are practicing in class, you can always focus on your breath, noticing how the different poses affect your ability to breathe, or you can pay special attention to how your teacher's specific alignment cues affect your body as a whole. Does making a small change somewhere ripple through your entire body?

Hold poses longer. Try holding poses for longer periods of time than you usually do. Notice the resistance that comes up in your body (as well as your mind). Also notice how the sensations in your body change with your time in the pose. Is there any new gripping or any new letting go?

Change your routine. If you do practice at home and realize that you have been practicing your poses on autopilot, try doing something different. For example, practice on the left side first instead of the right. How does that feel? Or do all of your twisting poses, even all the standing poses, without turning your head. Notice how hard that is and how different your neck feels. Try using props if you never have and see what kind of difference it makes. Or if you use props regularly, try a different height (lower or higher) or try practicing without props and see how that feels.

BREATH PRACTICES FOR EQUANIMITY

When Debbie Cabusas added breath practices (*pranayama*) to her regular yoga practice, she noticed some surprising changes. In addition to eliminating her sugar cravings—which helped her lose thirty pounds—her regular pranayama practice reduced her blood pressure levels and lowered her resting heart rate, increased her lung capacity, and helped her become noticeably calmer. She says, "I am happier and more accepting of and compassionate with myself and others. I appreciate my life."[8]

Yoga breath practices allow you to self-regulate. When you need soothing, you can use calming breath practices. When you need uplifting or energizing, you can use stimulating breath practices. And when you need just a moderate amount of calming or stimulating, you can use balancing practices.

Like the breath awareness practice described in chapter 9, structured breath practices require quite a bit of concentration and are a good way to take your mind off regrets about the past, worries about the future, or negative reactions to the present. However, they work quite differently from simple breath awareness, which is why not all breath practices are relaxing.

Pranayama is more powerful than simple breath awareness because it provides you with a key to your nervous system. While you cannot tell your nervous system directly to slow your heartbeat, digest your food more quickly, or start relaxing right this minute, you can control your breath. Even though you breathe without thinking about it, you can intentionally hold your breath, speed up your breath, slow down your breath, breathe through one nostril instead of the other, and so on.

This ability to alter your breathing is what provides you with some control over your nervous system's "involuntary functions." It's all due to the relationship between your heart and lungs and the nerves between them. With each breath you take, during your inhalation the nerves stimulate your heart to beat a little faster, and during your exhalation the nerves stimulate your heart to slow down a bit. So when you make one part of your breath cycle longer than the other, and you do this for several minutes, the accumulated effects change your heart rate, and that in turn changes the state of your entire nervous system.

Stimulating Practices

When you make your inhalations longer than your exhalations, for example, by using a two-second inhalation and a one-second exhalation, and you maintain that pattern for several minutes, your heart rate will speed up a bit. This increased heart rate sends a feedback message to your brain that your circumstances require activity, stimulating your stress response to prepare you physically and mentally to take action. So pranayama practices that lengthen your inhalation are practices you might want to do if you need energizing or are feeling depressed or lethargic. You would want to avoid them if you are feeling hyper, stressed out, anxious, or are suffering from insomnia.

Calming Practices

When you make your exhalations longer than your inhalations, for example, by using a one-second inhalation and a two-second exhalation or humming on your exhalation with a Bhramari breath, and you maintain that pattern for several minutes, your heart rate slows down a bit. This decreased rate sends a feedback message to your brain that your circumstances are more peaceful and calm now, which triggers the relaxation response, switching you into the rest-and-digest state.

So you may want to do pranayama practices that lengthen your exhalations if you are feeling hyper, stressed out, anxious, or are suffering from insomnia. Since most of us are not typically "understressed," about the only time you'd want to avoid these practices is when you are falling asleep and don't want to.

Balancing Practices

When you make your inhalations and your exhalations the same length, for example, by using a two-second inhalation with a two-second exhalation or by practicing alternate nostril breathing, you are only very subtly affecting your nervous system, maybe only slightly stimulating or calming it (depending on your current state).

These practices are good for times when you feel like you need "balancing" more than calming or stimulating or for when you wish to do a formal breath practice that will harness your mind to the present moment without having a strong effect on your nervous system.

HOW TO PRACTICE PRANAYAMA

This section contains detailed instructions for practicing the stimulating, calming, and balancing breath practices that we recommend. The practices we've chosen are generally considered safe for beginners as well as experienced practitioners (although you should never let yourself get short of breath). However, if you are a beginner who is interested in seriously exploring this branch of yoga, we recommend that you study with a trained teacher.

You can practice these in any comfortable seated position on the floor or on a chair (see "Choose Your Position" above) or in a reclined position where your chest is supported, such as version 4 of Reclined Cobbler's Pose or Relaxation Pose with similar support.

CAUTIONS: Anyone with active asthma should avoid all of these breath practices. If you are on medication and stable, however, you could give them a try, stopping immediately if they cause any breathing problems. Since all the practices require breathing through your nose, if you're congested due to illness or allergy, you should skip them until you can breathe normally.

STIMULATING BREATH PRACTICES

If you need uplifting or energizing—or if you tend to be lethargic in general—you can do any of the stimulating breath practices presented here. In addition, two of the practices—inhalation lengthening and inhalation pausing—can improve your ability to breathe, increasing your "vital capacity" and fostering respiratory system health (a large vital capacity is associated with excellent lung function).

CAUTION: With all of these breath practices, you are activating your stress response. So while these practices are good for times when you feel tired or sluggish, they are not recommended for people with anxiety, anxiety-based depression, or sleeping problems due to an overactive nervous system. Even if you're not suffering from anxiety or depression, if the practices make you feel agitated or even just unpleasant, stop practicing. You can use a balancing practice instead or stay with calming breath practices.

Lengthening Your Inhalation

With this practice, you gradually extend your inhalation, aiming for a 2:1 breath ratio, with your inhalation twice as long as your exhalation. If you can't comfortably manage a 2:1 breath ratio yet, simply practice an inhalation that is at your comfortable maximum. Always practice by breathing through your nose.

1. Practice simple breath awareness (see page 146) for one or two minutes. Without changing your breath, count the natural length of your inhalations and exhalations in seconds to see which part of your breath is longer, your inhalation or your exhalation.
2. Now you're going to lengthen your inhalation. If your inhalation is shorter than your exhalation, consciously make both parts of your breath last the same number of seconds by making your inhalation as long as your exhalation. As an example, let's say that your inhalation is naturally around two seconds, while your exhalation is around three seconds. To practice an equal breath, you would make both your inhalation and exhalation three seconds long.

   If your inhalation is already the same length as or longer than your exhalation, increase your inhalation by one second. For example, if your inhalation and exhalation are both around two seconds, you would lengthen your inhalation to three seconds.
3. If this is comfortable, continue for four rounds. If this is not comfortable, you could try increasing by half a second instead

(approximately the length of a one-syllable word). After four rounds, if you feel ready, you can proceed to the next step of increasing by another second or half a second. If this seems like it's going to be too much, simply continue with the last comfortable maximum for four more cycles and then return to step 1.

4. Try adding another second or half a second to your inhalation for four rounds of breath. If you've now reached a proportion of 2:1 (your inhalation is twice as long as your exhalation), this is your maximum. Practice your 2:1 breath for about a minute.

   If you have not yet reached a proportion of 2:1 and you are still comfortable, try lengthening your inhalation by another second or half a second for four rounds. Proceed in this fashion until you either reach a 2:1 ratio or pass your comfortable maximum. If you reach your 2:1 ratio, practice for one minute. However, if you pass your comfortable maximum, step back to your comfortable maximum and have that be your practice.

5. Now, start reversing the process by dropping one second or half a second for four rounds at a time. For example, if you were practicing a four-second inhalation, you'd return to three seconds for four rounds of breath. Continue in this way until you reach the length you started with in step 1, practicing that for four rounds.

6. Return to your natural breath and practice simple breath awareness for one to two minutes. Make a note of your comfortable maximum for the day and gradually work toward extending its length over time.

Skull Shining Breath (*Kapalabhati Pranayama*)

Traditionally, Skull Shining Breath is recommended for making you more present and alert, with a sharper mind. This is a stimulating breath practice that can wake you up if you're feeling sleepy or energize you when you're feeling sluggish. However, because it is a demanding practice, people who are tired may find it exhausting and should practice simple lengthening of the inhalation instead.

Technique

The basic breath technique consists of a quick, forceful exhalation through your nose followed by a quiet, natural inhalation, typically short, also through your nose. To make the quick, forceful exhalation, quickly contract your abdominal muscles toward your spine as you breathe out. (Imagine you have a down feather stuck to the opening of your nose, and you are trying to forcefully blow it off your nose.) This forceful exhalation should be loud enough to hear clearly. To take the natural inhalation, relax your belly and passively allow your breath to fill your lungs, without attempting to slow it. This soft inhalation should be much quieter—if at all audible—than your exhalation.

1. Practice simple breath awareness (see page 146) for one or two minutes.

2. About halfway through a natural exhalation, begin your first quick, forceful exhalation as described above. Follow the exhalation immediately with your quiet, natural inhalation and then pause gently at the end of your inhalation. On your next exhalation, begin with the quick, forceful exhalation for your first full cycle of Skull Shining Breath.

3. If you're new to the practice, acclimate to this style of breathing by starting with twelve to sixteen breaths. Keep your pace relaxed and relatively comfortable, ensuring that you don't feel short of breath, lightheaded, nauseated, or dizzy. Use the gentle pause at the end of the inhalation to slow your pace if necessary. If you experience any problems, return to normal breathing for a few minutes. If your symptoms fully resolve and you are back to feeling normal, you could then try one more cycle of twelve to sixteen breaths. If you rest and don't feel completely back to normal, skip the practice today and try it another day.

4. On your last breath cycle, contract your abdominal muscles toward your spine and squeeze all the breath out of your lungs with a long exhalation instead of a short one. Then take a gentle full inhalation followed by a natural, relaxed exhalation.

5. Take a short break of about one minute and return to your natural breathing pattern. Then, if you feel up to it, repeat a second set of twelve to sixteen breaths.

6. Eventually, over time, work up to two sets of sixty repetitions, with a short break of about one minute between the sets. As you get more accustomed to the practice, you can also speed up your breath quite a bit by shortening or eliminating the pauses, practicing up to two cycles per second.

7. When you have completed two cycles, return to your natural breath and practice simple breath awareness for one to two minutes. Notice whether you feel more alert, mentally clear, and/or enlivened.

CALMING BREATH PRACTICES

All of our calming breath practices allow you to reduce stress levels, soothe yourself, and quiet your mind and nervous system. In addition, two of these practices, exhalation pausing and exhalation lengthening, can improve your ability to breathe, increasing your "vital capacity" (a large vital capacity is associated with excellent lung function) and fostering respiratory system health.

You are activating your relaxation response with these breath practices, so while they are good for times when you are looking for quieting or calming, if they make you feel too sluggish or heavy, you can use a balancing practice instead (see "Balancing Breath Practices" on page 179). If they make you feel agitated or unpleasant, just stop practicing.

Exhalation Lengthening

With this practice, you gradually extend your exhalation, aiming for a 1:2 breath ratio, with your exhalation twice as long as your inhalation. If you can't comfortably practice a 1:2 breath ratio at this time, simply practice an exhalation that is at your comfortable maximum. Always practice by breathing through your nose.

1. Practice simple breath awareness (page 146) for one or two minutes. Without changing your breath, count the natural length of your inhalations and exhalations in seconds to see which part of your breath is longer, your inhalation or your exhalation.
2. Now you're going to lengthen your exhalation. If your exhalation is shorter than your inhalation, consciously make both parts of your breath last the same number of seconds by making your exhalation as long as your inhalation. As an example, let's say that your exhalation is naturally around two seconds, while your inhalation is around three seconds. To practice an equal breath, you would make both your inhalation and exhalation three seconds long.
3. If your exhalation is already the same length as or longer than your inhalation, increase your exhalation by one second. For example, if your inhalation and exhalation are both around two seconds, you would lengthen your exhalation to three seconds.
4. If this is comfortable, continue for four rounds. If this is not comfortable, you could try increasing by half a second instead (approximately the length of a one-syllable word). After four rounds, if you feel ready, you can proceed to the next step of increasing by another second or half a second. If this seems like it's going to be too much,

simply continue with your last comfortable maximum for four more cycles and then return to step 1.

5. Try adding another second or half a second to your exhalation for four rounds of breath. If you've now reached a ratio of 1:2 (your exhalation is twice as long as your inhalation), this is your maximum. Practice your 1:2 breath for about a minute.

6. If you have not yet reached a proportion of 1:2 and you are still comfortable, try lengthening your exhalation by another second or half a second for four rounds. Proceed in this fashion until you either reach a 1:2 ratio or pass your comfortable maximum. If you reach your 1:2 ratio, continue practicing at that ratio as described below. However, if you are not comfortable, step back to your comfortable maximum and have that be your practice.

7. After reaching a comfortable 1:2 ratio (or your comfortable maximum), you can continue to practice at this level for two to three minutes. Over time, you can gradually work up to five minutes. If at any time your breath becomes labored or uncomfortable in any way or you start feeling agitated or panicky, stop and return to your natural breath.

8. To gradually return to your natural breath, start reversing the process by dropping one second or half a second for four rounds at a time. For example, if you were practicing a four-second exhalation, you'd return to three seconds for four rounds of breath. Continue in this way until you reach the length you started with in step 1 and practice that for four rounds.

9. Return to your natural breath and practice simple breath awareness for one to two minutes. Make a note of your comfortable maximum for the day and gradually work toward extending its length over time.

Another way to lengthen your exhalation to a 1:2 ratio is to use a gentle version of *ujjayi* breathing for your exhalation only. To do this, breathe in normally through your nose, with a relaxed feeling in your throat and vocal cords. Then, as you start to exhale, slightly constrict your throat, keeping it very gentle and relatively quiet. This action in your throat is similar to the one some people use when they breathe on their glasses to clean them, and it will naturally slow down your exhalation a bit and bring you closer to a 1:2 ratio.

Exhalation Pausing

At the end of each inhalation, your breath naturally pauses, very briefly, before your exhalation begins. Likewise, at the end of your exhalation, there's a brief pause before your next inhalation begins. So every breath cycle naturally has four stages: inhalation, pause, exhalation, pause.

With exhalation pausing, you consciously lengthen the pause after your exhalation for a given amount of time, sometimes for a brief moment and other times for one, two, or three seconds (or more, in more advanced practices). This pausing should be a soft suspension of your breath, not a gripped "holding" as you might do holding your breath underwater.

Lengthening the pause at the end of the exhalation can enhance the calming effects of a longer exhalation. In addition, lengthening the pause may help strengthen your breathing muscles.

The instructions we're providing are for adding an exhalation pause to an equal breath. However, you can combine exhalation pausing with extended exhalations (described above). If you do, your maximum pause should be the length of your inhalation. Always practice by breathing through your nose.

1. Start by practicing equal inhalations and exhalations, as described under "Equal Breath" on page 130. In our example, we'll assume you're practicing a two-second inhalation and a two-second exhalation. Continue for four rounds of breath.

2. On your next round of breath, gently lengthen the pause after your exhalation to half a second (or the length of a one-syllable word). If this is comfortable, continue for four rounds. After four rounds, if you feel ready, you can proceed to the next step of increasing your pause to a second. If this seems like it's going to be too much, simply continue at your comfortable maximum for four more cycles and then return to step 1.

3. Try lengthening the pause to one full second for four rounds of breath. If this is still comfortable, lengthen by another half a second, proceeding in this fashion until your pauses are either equal to the length of your inhalations and exhalations or you have passed your comfortable maximum. For example, if you are breathing two-second inhalations and exhalations, stop when you have reached two-second pauses. But if your comfortable maximum is one-and-a-half seconds, step back to that timing for your practice.

4. Once you reach your comfortable maximum, you can continue to practice at this level for two to three minutes, working up to five minutes over time. If at any time your breath becomes labored or uncomfortable in any way, or you start feeling agitated or panicky, stop and return to your natural breath.

5. Return to your natural breath and practice simple breath awareness

for one to two minutes. Make a note of your comfortable maximum for pausing for the day and gradually work toward extending its length over time.

Buzzing Bee Breath (Bhramari Pranayama)

In this breath practice, you make a buzzing sound as you exhale, which naturally lengthens your exhalation and creates a calming effect. Always practice by breathing through your nose.

1. Practice simple breath awareness (page 146) for one or two minutes.
2. Inhale normally through your nose. Then, keeping your mouth closed, make a low- to medium-pitched humming or buzzing sound in your throat as you exhale. As you make the sound—which should last the entire length of your exhalation—sense the vibration of the sound waves in your throat and even in your skull and brain.
3. After you complete your exhalation, inhale through your nose.
4. If you're comfortable, repeat the cycle. Try to make the transitions in and out of your exhalations smooth and even. If at any time your breath becomes labored or uncomfortable in any way, or you start feeling agitated or panicky, stop and return to your natural breath.
5. Start with twelve to sixteen rounds of Buzzing Bee Breath, for approximately one minute, and work up to two- to three-minute practices over time.
6. Return to your natural breath and practice simple breath awareness for one to two minutes. Notice whether this practice was quieting and calming or had other effects on you.

BALANCING BREATH PRACTICES

When you need just a moderate amount of calming or stimulating, you can use balancing practices. With a balancing breath, such as when you make your inhalations and your exhalations the same length or practice alternate nostril breathing, you are only subtly affecting your nervous system, slightly stimulating or calming it (depending on your current state).

So these breath practices are good for times when you feel like you need "balancing," such as in the morning when you first wake up and want just a bit of stimulation or when you've just left work and want a bit of calming. If you're anxious and having mild breathing problems, practicing an equal breath can help you get your breathing back under control, making it more steady and even. The gradual lengthening of equal breath practice (below) can improve your ability to breathe, increasing your vital capacity and promoting a healthy respiratory system.

You can also use these practices when you wish to do a formal breath practice that will harness your mind to the present moment without having a strong effect on your nervous system.

Equal Breath (*Sama Vritti*)

Always practice by breathing through your nose.

1. Practice simple breath awareness (page 146) for one or two minutes. Without changing your breath, count the natural length of your inhalations and exhalations in seconds to see which part of your breath is longer, your inhalation or exhalation.
2. Consciously make both parts of your breath last the same length of time by making the longer part the same number of seconds as the shorter part. As an example, let's say that your inhalation is naturally around three seconds, while your exhalation is around two seconds. To practice an equal breath, you would make both your inhalation and exhalation two seconds long.
3. Practice for two to three minutes or twenty-four to thirty-six rounds. If your breath becomes labored or uncomfortable in any way, or you start feeling agitated or panicky, stop and return to your natural breath.
4. When your practice is complete, return to your natural breath and practice simple breath awareness for one to two minutes.

Gradual Lengthening of Equal Breath

Always practice by breathing through your nose.

1. Start by practicing equal inhalations and exhalations, as described above, for four rounds of breath. In our example, we'll assume you're practicing a two-second inhalation and a two-second exhalation. Continue for four rounds of breath.
2. Add one second to both your inhalation and exhalation. If this is comfortable, continue for four rounds. If this is not comfortable, try increasing by half a second instead (approximately the length of a one-syllable word) or return to step 1 and have that be your practice. After four rounds, if you feel ready, proceed to the next step of increasing by another second. If this seems like it's going to be too much, simply continue with your last comfortable maximum for four more cycles and then return to step 1.

3. Try adding another second to your inhalation and exhalation for four rounds of breath. If this is still comfortable, lengthen both by another second, proceeding in this fashion until you pass your comfortable maximum. For example, when you attempt a six-second practice, you might realize that you can only comfortably inhale for five seconds while exhaling for six seconds, or vice versa. At this point, step back to your comfortable maximum and repeat for four more cycles. For example, if you found that a six-second breath practice was too much, you would step back to a five-second breath for four rounds.

4. Now, start reversing the process by dropping one second for four rounds. For example, if you were practicing for five seconds, you'd return to four seconds for four rounds of breath. Continue in this way until you reach the length you started with in step 1 and practice that for four rounds.

5. Return to your natural breath and practice simple breath awareness for one to two minutes. Make a note of your comfortable maximum for the day and gradually work toward extending its length over time.

Alternate Nostril Breathing (*Nadi Sodhana*)

With this breath practice, you breathe through one nostril at a time, alternating between sides with each exhalation. The classic way to do this is by using your right hand to gently close the nostril you're not using, typically using your right thumb to close your right nostril and your right ring and pinky fingers to close your left nostril. But there are many different hand positions that you can use for this practice. Feel free to use any other method you've been taught.

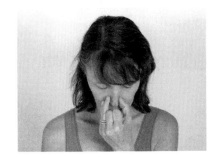

1. Practice simple breath awareness (page 146) for one or two minutes.
2. With your left hand relaxed in your lap, bring your right hand in front of your face with your palm facing your head and your fingers facing directly up. Curl your index finger and middle finger toward your palm. Then gently rest your thumb on your right nostril and your ring and pinky fingers on your left nostril (don't block either nostril yet).
3. Inhale and exhale completely through both nostrils.
4. Pause and gently close your right nostril with your thumb.
5. Inhale through your left nostril.
6. Pause and gently close your left nostril with your ring and pinky fingers and open your right nostril. Exhale through your right nostril.
7. Inhale through your right nostril.

8. Pause and gently close your right nostril with your thumb and open your left nostril. Exhale through your left nostril. You have now completed one cycle of nadi sodhana.

9. Repeat the cycle six to twelve times. If at any time your breath becomes labored or uncomfortable in any way, or you start feeling agitated or panicky, stop and return to your natural breath.

10. Finish on an exhalation through your left nostril, release your hand, and return to your natural breath.

11. Practice simple breath awareness for one to two minutes.

ASANAS AND YOUR EMOTIONS

For many people, yoga poses and practices can have a strong effect on their moods and emotions. This is something you should take into consideration when you practice on your own. Knowing how certain poses will affect you will not only help you choose which poses to do at a particular time of day but also which poses to practice to balance your emotions and self-regulate (see page 184).

In this section we're grouping the yoga poses into general categories, and for each category, we'll list some of the typical emotional effects. In the end, however, don't just take our word for it. You should always rely on your personal experience to guide you. We once had a student who said that twists made her sleepy. That's not the traditional view of how twists affect us, but if this woman felt they made her sleepy, well, then that's what they did!

Standing poses. These are considered to be very grounding poses, which immediately engage your body-mind and bring you into the present moment. So they are good poses to do when you are worried, distracted, or agitated. Standing poses are also stimulating, because being upright raises your blood pressure and increases your heart rate (the opposite of being inverted). So while these are great poses to do in the morning or afternoon, these are not good poses to do before bedtime if you have trouble sleeping.

Dynamic poses and flow sequences. Poses that are linked together with the breath, including Sun Salutations, moving dynamically between Mountain Pose to Standing Forward Bend, or even moving from Mountain Pose to Arms Overhead Pose and back, can energize your emotional body and help lift you out of lethargy, depression, or sadness. Like standing poses, dynamic poses and flow sequences are stimulating. So while these practices are great in the morning or afternoon, they are not good to do before bedtime if you have trouble sleeping.

Backbends. These poses are considered to be energizing and uplifting. They may help create more energy when you are tired and lift you out of depression or sadness. On the negative side, they may actually make you too hyper if you are already nervous, and some people have difficulty falling asleep after practicing backbends. Because they literally open the heart area, they may cause strong emotions to arise—some people find themselves crying after doing a lot of backbends. One way to access the energizing, uplifting quality of these poses without overstimulating yourself is to do passive, supported backbends, such as Supported Backbend and the supported versions of Bridge Pose.

Twists. These poses are considered to be cleansing. They can help release stress from your body-mind. On the negative side, twists may also release difficult feelings or emotions, so they may actually leave you feeling a bit uncomfortable emotionally.

Forward bends. These poses are considered to be quieting, introverted poses. They can calm you down when you are feeling agitated or hyper and help you rest when you are feeling fatigued. On the negative side, the inward-turning quality of the poses may cause you to brood or feel claustrophobic. Supported versions that remove the physical resistance from these poses, such as version 4 of Seated Forward Bend, can be extremely quieting and calming for those who like them.

Inverted poses. These poses are considered to be soothing and centering. Because they are so effective for triggering the relaxation response, we've dedicated an entire section of the book to them (see "Supported Inverted Poses" on page 152). And because they don't seem to cause any brooding or claustrophobia the way forward bends do for some, they're especially beneficial for anxiety and depression. If they work for you, you can include them in any type of practice, active or restorative, or even practice the poses on their own.

Balance pose. These poses are considered to be demanding and require a lot of mental focus. Because they completely engage your minds they can help distract you from concerns outside the yoga room. This may lift your spirits or at least give you a break from your obsessions. If standing balance poses are easy for you, try arm balances. Side Plank Pose counts as one!

Hip openers and seated poses. These poses are considered to be very grounding and centering. They seem to release tension, especially from your legs, and bring you into the present moment. On the negative side, opening the hips can sometimes feel emotionally uncomfortable, so you might not feel up to doing them on some days.

SELF-REGULATION: MONITORING AND MANAGING YOUR INTERNAL STATES

According to a recent scientific study, all eight branches of yoga are complementary tools that allow you to improve your ability to "self-regulate." Nina says that although "self-regulation" is a new concept to her, when she learned about it, she realized right away that because she's been practicing yoga for over twenty years to reduce her stress levels, to restore her when she's depleted, to energize her when she's fatigued, and to uplift her when she's feeling a bit depressed, she's been self-regulating all this time without even knowing it.

Self-regulation involves monitoring and managing your internal states. You understand what the state of being calm and alert feels like, and you know which activities draw you out of that state and which activities (including yoga practices) return you to it. Self-regulation also includes the ability to comfort yourself when you are worried or anxious and to cheer yourself up when you're feeling blue.

Naturally, being able to self-regulate, rather than reacting impulsively as a result of emotions such as anger or fear, contributes to your overall equanimity. Self-regulation also enables you to act in your long-term interest and consistent with your deepest values rather than impulsively.

The term "self-regulation" is often used to describe children (you can imagine what a child who is not able to self-regulate might be like), but it can apply to everyone because who among us is not sometimes swamped with emotions that cause us to do things we might later regret?

To help explain exactly how yoga can help you to self-regulate, we have broken the process down into the following five phases:

1. Monitoring your internal states—Whether you are meditating or practicing poses mindfully, using your witness mind as we described above allows you to observe your emotional responses and thought patterns, helping you uncover habitual responses to stressors. This is the first step toward improving self-regulation.

2. Understanding what it feels like to be calm and alert—Yoga practices that trigger the relaxation response allow you to experience conscious relaxation in the safety of the yoga room. In this state, your mind opens to a wider range of possible reactions to stressors.

Having this experience in the yoga room teaches you that you can learn to respond to stressors in the real world in a similar way.

3. Recognizing when certain activities help you return to those states most easily—Experimenting with a wide range of yoga practices, including yoga poses, relaxation techniques, meditation techniques, and breath techniques, and even studying yoga philosophy helps you recognize which yoga "activities" work best to help you return to a more balanced state.

4. Recognizing what draws you out of those states—Working with your witness mind in the yoga room trains you to start observing yourself in more volatile situations in your everyday life. You can learn which external or internal events set you off or make you feel out of balance. Some of these may be things you can change, such as by eating more regularly, finding a less stressful way to get to work, or getting more sleep. For stressors you can't avoid, you can learn to respond differently to them by practicing stress management techniques to dial down stress levels.

5. Managing your internal states—In addition to using yoga poses and breath practices for relaxation, you can use them to energize yourself when you're feeling fatigued and to uplift yourself when you're feeling depressed. Using yoga to manage your internal states allows you to make yourself feel better through your own efforts rather than relying on outside events or other people to calm you down or cheer you up, and it gives you a sense of control over your emotional life.

A BEAUTIFUL INNER SUPPORT SYSTEM

Although our equanimity practices are very effective for supporting us in the present, allowing us to let go of regrets about the past and worries about the future and to face challenges in the here and now with a sense of balance, practicing regularly will also help prepare us for challenges we may face in the future. So even though it can be tempting to use your equanimity practices on an as-needed basis, we recommend you practice regularly even during "easeful" times, so that those practices will be available to you as a "beautiful inner support system" whenever you need them.

A longtime practitioner of both Buddhist meditation and yoga, Jill Satterfield practiced pretty much daily, with meditation, asanas, and pranayama all playing a part. She saw all of those practices show their strength for her when she endured a couple of years of uncertainty after being

Sometimes we don't fully appreciate the progress or importance of our practices, but there will be a time when our practices show up and show their strength and depth. So practicing both in the times that are easeful and in the times that are not creates this beautiful inner support system that is there for us when things get really rough.

— Jill Satterfield, "Recovering from Heart Surgery," from the *Yoga for Healthy Aging* blog diagnosed with a heart defect and being told she would "know" when the time was right for surgery, and then going through the surgery itself. She says they helped her because after many years of being mindful of her thoughts, emotions, and the sensations in her body, she developed a keen sense of what could be beneficial and when something was too much or too soon. She also said:

> Having meditated for thirty years, my meditation practice showed up the most as far as supporting me in the pre-surgery stage. I wasn't afraid, I wasn't anxious, I wasn't angry; I was surprisingly okay with the reality of my situation. My mind, and the training of my mind—of being in the present and not far-flung into the unknown future of fear and anxiety—really was a great blessing. I was at ease with what was happening and that was great considering it went on for two years.[9]

That to us is the very essence of equanimity.

Yoga Philosophy

YOGA PHILOSOPHY INCLUDES WISDOM THAT CAN CHANGE YOUR entire perspective on life. As we said in chapter 1, the original aim of yoga was peace of mind, and the yoga texts were written to guide us toward that goal. In fact, the yoga texts are so full of profound observations about the nature of the mind and the causes of suffering that you are sure to find something that speaks to you. Mohandas K. Gandhi said that the wisdom of the Bhagavad Gita allowed him to maintain peace of mind as he fought for social justice. Ralph Waldo Emerson was inspired by early translations of yogic texts as he developed his philosophy of transcendentalism. Henry David Thoreau practiced meditation and pondered yogic concepts as he explored the nature of solitude during his time at Walden Pond. He wrote in an 1849 letter to his friend H. G. O. Blake:

> Depend upon it that, rude and careless as I am, I would fain practice the *yoga* faithfully.
>
> "The yogi, absorbed in contemplation, contributes in his degree to creation: he breathes a divine perfume, he hears wonderful things. Divine forms traverse him without tearing him, and, united to the nature which is proper to him, he goes, he acts as animating original matter."
>
> To some extent, and at rare intervals, even I am a yogi.[1]

Hear now the wisdom of Yoga, path of the Eternal and freedom from bondage.

No step is lost on this path, and no dangers are found. And even a little progress is freedom from fear.

— Juan Mascaró, translator,
The Bhagavad Gita

Even in modern times, the wisdom of yoga can be your guiding light. After a stint in rehab for alcohol and drug abuse, Evelyn Zak's sponsor took her to a yoga class. She wasn't sure about going but had decided to do whatever was suggested by the people she trusted to keep her from relapsing. That first class led her to regular practice, then more intensive studies, and eventually she trained to be a yoga teacher and yoga therapist. Now she's been alcohol and drug free for thirty years, and she says that although all the branches of yoga were helpful in keeping her sober, the yogic concept of *ahimsa* (nonviolence) was just what the doctor ordered. She explains it this way:

> If the concept of ahimsa is that to hurt another being is the same as hurting oneself, then it stands to reason that to hurt oneself is to hurt another being. Anyone who has dealt with addiction, either as a patient or a support person, knows that everyone gets hurt at some level.[2]

These days Evelyn works as a yoga therapist and substance abuse counselor, sharing yogic principles with children, seniors, preachers, Rotary Clubs, problem gamblers, large groups of lawyers, marathon runners, people with disabilities, people with eating disorders, and more. She says:

> If I hadn't absorbed the concept of ahimsa along the way, I don't believe any of this would have been possible because I wouldn't have been in a position to learn and absorb and I wouldn't have cared enough about anyone else to share what I found to be so personally valuable.[3]

Studying yoga philosophy provides you with an alternative way of thinking about your life, enabling you to be more content with what you have and what you don't have and to become more comfortable with change. The yoga texts also provide insights into the nature of the mind that you can use to change your mental habits and behavior patterns. Studying the philosophy is as much a part of yoga as any of the other practices, and it is available to anyone, regardless of age or physical condition.

For this book, we came up with a list of essential yoga concepts we believe will assist you in cultivating equanimity. We intentionally kept this list limited in order to keep it manageable (not because we think this list covers everything valuable in the yoga texts).

PRACTICE

What a difference there is between reading a bunch of wise words in an ancient yoga text—or any book for that matter—and actually living wisely! Many years ago, when she was suffering from stress-related anxiety, Nina's therapist said to her, "Stop worrying so much." It's almost funny now, but at the time, Nina was horrified (and never went back to see that therapist). Well, yes, she needed to stop worrying so much, but hearing the words *stop worrying* wasn't exactly helpful, as you might imagine.

How do we move from being inspired by words of wisdom to incorporating wisdom into our daily lives? In the Bhagavad Gita, Arjuna asks Krishna this very question:

> "You have taught that the essence of yoga
> is equanimity, Krishna;
> but since the mind is so restless,
> how can that be achieved?
>
> The mind is restless, unsteady,
> turbulent, wild, stubborn;
> truly, it seems to me
> as hard to master as the wind."

Krishna replies:

> "You are right, Arjuna: the mind
> is restless and hard to master;
> but by constant practice and detachment
> it *can* be mastered in the end."[4]

Everything we want to do well takes practice and that includes achieving the goals we set for our yoga practice. Whether these goals are cultivating equanimity, changing the way you react to stress, meditating to quiet your mind, or just improving balance or strength, practicing is the only path that will get you there. Around 800 years later, The Yoga Sutras expanded on this concept of practice by saying that practice should be diligent, combined with unattached awareness (detachment), and pursued with "eagerness, sincerity, and continuity" for a long time. In *Yoga Sūtras of Patañjali*, Edwin Bryant says that maintaining a garden is a useful metaphor for the practice of yoga because, "As any gardener knows, maintaining a garden takes devotion and uninterrupted weeding and pest control for a prolonged period of time."[5]

Practice becomes firmly established when it has been cultivated uninterruptedly and with devotion over a prolonged period of time.

—Sutra 1.14, translated by Edwin F. Bryant

Although these original recommendations were specifically for quieting the mind (the goal of yoga in The Yoga Sutras), they apply whatever your goal is. So keep that in mind every time you take your first steps on a new path for cultivating well-being, whether physical, emotional, or spiritual.

Of course, it's easy enough to imagine diligently practicing strengthening poses to foster physical strength, stress management practices to reduce chronic stress, or equanimity practices to balance your emotions. But how do you diligently practice wisdom?

Unfortunately, we all have habitual patterns of thought and ways of reacting to challenges that are hard to change. You might say we're stuck in some serious ruts! As a matter of fact, ancient yogis even had a word for these thought and behavior patterns: *samskaras* (impressions). They said that with every thought we have and action we take we leave samskaras on "the hot wax of the mind." These impressions get deeper and deeper with repetition. In his book *The Wisdom of Yoga,* psychologist Stephen Cope actually describes samskaras as "ruts":

> Samskāras are like little tracks, little vectors, little ruts in the muddy road. The next time the car travels that road, these muddy ruts will have hardened into permanent fixtures, and the car wheels will want to slide into them. Indeed it's easier to steer right into them than to try to avoid them.[6]

It takes diligent practice combined with detachment to avoid these ruts and change your mental habits! The first step is to observe your mental habits with unattached awareness. As you meditate, practice yoga mindfully, and go about your everyday life, notice the habitual way your mind works, without judgment. For example, as Nina worked with her tendency toward anxiety, she observed a pattern of worrying about the future, even about events that might not even happen. For fun, she called her rut "panicking too soon."

The second step is to use the wisdom of yoga to respond with a more helpful reaction or thought. Sutra 2.33 of The Yoga Sutras recommends practicing *pratipaksha bhavanam*, which means "cultivating the opposite" or "cultivating counteracting thoughts":

> Upon being harassed by negative thoughts, one should cultivate counteracting thoughts.[7]

This could mean consciously thinking with compassion about someone you dislike or about yourself when you feel self-hatred or cultivating gratitude for the good things in your life when you feel unhappy with your current circumstances. For Nina, this meant that every time she would catch herself spiraling into anxiety, she would remind herself there was another way to respond to stressful situations by reciting this stanza from the Bhagavad Gita:

> Self-possessed, resolute, act
> without any thought of results,
> open to success or failure.
> This equanimity is yoga.[8]

Our colleague Elizabeth Ann Gibbs recommends writing down your counteracting thought and taping it to the fridge or bathroom mirror so it's visible every day and then repeating it often, silently or out loud, as you move through your yoga practice or even through your day. That way, it will be mentally handy when you notice yourself slipping back into your old ruts. She says that over time and with practice this technique enables you to transform an unhealthy reaction into a positive, productive response.

As Nina continued practicing this technique, she eventually noticed that the more often she responded to stress by reminding herself that she could let go of thoughts of results, the easier it became. She felt that cultivating this new habit was like exercising an initially weak muscle that got stronger and stronger over time. You can also think of it as creating a new, positive samskara to replace the old one. Using his garden metaphor, Edwin Byrant compares negative thoughts to weeds and positive thoughts to flowers:

> As in a garden, the more one makes an effort to uproot weeds, the more the bed will eventually become a receptacle for fragrant flowers, which will then grow and reseed of their own accord until there is hardly any room for the weeds to surface.[9]

DETACHMENT

Most people don't realize that the most famous yogi of the twentieth century was Mohandas K. Gandhi. What made him a great yogi wasn't the number of Sun Salutations he did (not very many, if any at all) but his practice of yoga in action (karma yoga), inspired by the seminal yoga text the Bhagavad Gita, which he referred to as his "mother."

Written around 500 to 400 B.C.E., the Bhagavad Gita (the Gita) is one section of a much longer work, the Mahabharata. The Gita tells the story of Arjuna, a warrior in the Pandava army, who is in the middle of a battle.

In this wisdom, a man goes beyond what is well done and what is not well done. Go thou therefore to wisdom: Yoga is wisdom in work.

— Juan Mascaró, translator,
The Bhagavad Gita

(Gandhi, who was a proponent of nonviolence, believed that this battle was a metaphor for the "duel that perpetually goes on in the hearts of mankind.") When Arjuna sees the opposition, he comes to a sudden halt. Although in his view the Kavaras are corrupt rulers who seized the throne illegitimately, he sees esteemed teachers, elders, and relatives in the opposing army. So Arjuna tells Krishna, who is both his charioteer and friend, that he has decided not to fight. Krishna speaks to him about yoga (the entire Gita is their dialogue). In the end, Arjuna decides to return to the battle, taking the yogic approach to it that Krishna—who he learns is a Hindu deity—recommends. Here is what Krishna says to him:

> Set thy heart upon thy work, but never on its reward. Work not for a reward; but never cease to do thy work.
>
> Do thy work in the peace of Yoga and, free from selfish desires, be not moved in success or failure. Yoga is evenness of mind—a peace that is ever the same.[10]

Detachment here means that we do our work—whatever that is—without being attached to the outcome (reward) of our actions. That is how we can do what we need to do while at the same time staying calm and focused. This approach of letting go of all results, whether good or bad, and focusing on the action alone is the essence of yoga.

For Gandhi "work" meant fighting for the independence of India and the rights of the oppressed through nonviolent action. He describes the importance of doing work without attachment to results this way:

> He who is ever brooding over result often loses nerve in the performance of his duty. He becomes impatient and then gives vent to anger and begins to do unworthy things; he jumps from action to action never remaining faithful to any. He who broods over results is like a man given to objects of the senses; he is ever distracted, he says goodbye to all scruples, everything is right in his estimation and he therefore resorts to means fair and foul to attain his end.[11]

We introduced the concept of detachment in chapter 1 as our philosophy of yoga for healthy aging. We also mentioned the term in our section on practice because an integral aspect of practice is that it should be done with "unattached awareness." But this concept is as useful outside of the yoga room as it is inside it. For no matter what work we have to do, whether it is raising children, going to a 9-to-5 job, being politically active, or caretaking a family member, taking action without attachment to the outcome of our action allows us to do what we need to do and be at peace with the results.

Students often ask us, "If you don't care about whether you succeed or fail, why would you even bother taking actions?" In the Bhagavad Gita, Krishna actually answers this very same question:

> Action is greater than inaction: perform therefore thy task in life.
> Even the life of the body could not be if there were no action.[12]

Krishna tells Arjuna that action is a necessary part of human existence and that even the body can't exist without it. After all, we all have to get up in the morning, go to jobs, and take care of ourselves and our families, and some of us have a calling, whether it's to be a teacher, an artist, a scientist, or a social activist. The only way to attain equanimity is to do your work—whatever it is—without any thoughts of results, remaining open to success or failure.

The Yoga Sutras recommends practicing meditation itself with detachment (or unattached awareness). That's simply because worrying about whether your meditation practice is quieting your mind not only disturbs your equanimity in the moment but also makes it less likely that you'll succeed.

Other questions we frequently hear are, "Isn't it self-contradictory to have a goal but not be attached to whether or not you achieve it? How is it even a goal if you're not attached to the outcome?" It's important to make the distinction between caring about your work—doing something you feel passionate about—and being fixated on the results. Just think of the many types of work where even if you do the absolute best job you can, you may not be able to succeed. For example, picture a lawyer trying to help a client they believe is innocent, an emergency medical technician trying to save a life, or a teacher hoping to help a room full of students succeed in learning.

Although Gandhi did achieve his goal of Indian independence that he worked so long for, his final work was promoting religious harmony in newly independent India. In those efforts he did not succeed, and they eventually led to his death, as he was assassinated by a religious fanatic. But the wisdom of the Bhagavad Gita that he cultivated through his practice of nonattachment enabled him to do all of the work he believed in, whether he succeeded or failed. He said:

> What effect this reading of the Gita had on my friends only they
> can say but to me the Gita became an infallible guide of conduct.

It became my dictionary of daily reference. Just as I turned to the English dictionary for the meanings of English words that I did not understand, I turned to this dictionary of conduct for a ready solution to all my troubles and trials.[13]

QUIETING THE MIND

By watching my mind for so many years now, I've befriended impermanence and change. Stability in anything except awareness has gone off the wish list, which has made my life more full of ease. This is the sanity and ease of not knowing: being comfortable — not always liking, but being comfortable — with change.

— Jill Satterfield, "Spiritual Sanity" from the *Yoga for Healthy Aging* blog

Patanjali's Yoga Sutras is a classic yoga text from around 400 C.E. that describes the eight-fold path of yoga (Raja Yoga). It consists of 195 aphorisms (sutras), which were compiled from various other texts to provide an overview of yoga at the time. Unlike the Bhagavad Gita, The Yoga Sutras was not considered one of the major yoga texts prior to the twentieth century. However, in the late nineteenth century, Swami Vivekananda, who many credit with bringing yoga to the West, began heavily promoting it. Since then it has become one of the most popular of all the yoga texts, especially in the West. Although the sutras are short and easy to memorize, they also require quite a bit of unpacking!

Sutra 1.2 provides a basic definition of yoga, but various Sanskrit translators tend to translate this short definition quite differently. Let's start by looking at just one translation:

> *Yoga cittavritti nirodha*
> Yoga is the cessation of movements in the consciousness.[14]

This confuses many of us the first time we read it. What are the movements in the consciousness (cittavritti)? And why on earth would we want them to cease? This is the reason we like to share another more unusual translation of the sutra by Georg Feuerstein in his book *Yoga: The Technology of Ecstasy*, that translates *vritti* as "whirls" rather than movements or fluctuations:

> Patanjali defines Yoga simply as "the restriction of the whirls of consciousness."[15]

It turns out that the word *vritti* literally means "whirlpool." So you can think of vrittis as "whirlpools" of the mind. Have you ever noticed how your mind tends to whirl or cycle over and over with the same thoughts, especially when you are anxious, depressed, or mentally stressed out? For example, Nina Rook describes the anxiety she suffered before she started practicing yoga this way:

As a working mother, before that was commonplace in corporate life, there were uncertainties about parenting, childcare, work/life conflicts, and chipping away at the glass ceiling. I remember whole nights spent running the same loops of "what ifs."[16]

When we're worried or anxious, we tend to get caught up in concerns about the future: "What if I miss my deadline?" "What if the plane crashes?" "What if I can't fall asleep tonight?" When we're sad or depressed, we tend to get caught up in regrets about the past: "If only my lover hadn't left me." "If only my parents had loved me more." "If only I'd taken a different job." Our vrittis can also include judgments about the present: "I'm such a loser." "That person looks like a jerk." "This meditation session is a complete failure." Those little whirlpools are so powerful, they suck us right in.

According to The Yoga Sutras, quieting the mind—restricting all those regrets, worries, and judgments—allows you to experience the reality of the present moment and be comfortable with change as it unfolds.

When Jill Satterfield, introduced in chapter 8, noticed that her heart didn't seem to be beating properly and was working too hard all the time, she learned that a virus had burned away her mitral valve and created a hole in the wall between two of the chambers in her heart. Although she needed surgery to repair her heart, her doctors recommended that she wait until her symptoms worsened, saying she would know when the time was right. During that waiting period, her energy was low, her brain was foggy, and her muscles were always sore. Because she didn't feel normal or rested, she wasn't able to take on much work, as she never knew if she would need to sit or lie down or would be relatively okay. She had no idea how long this waiting period would last.

She says now that her longtime meditation allowed her to be "at ease" with all that uncertainty. Years of practice trained her mind to be able to focus on the present instead of being flung forward into an "unknown future of fear and anxiety." She calls this "spiritual sanity," and says:

> Freedom comes with the ability to be in the present and with not knowing or assuming or deciding what will come next, but riding the proverbial waves of natural moment-to-moment change.[17]

In The Yoga Sutras, quieting the mind through meditation is recommended as the antidote to the five afflictions, our reactions to life that are the source of our suffering:

The five afflictions which disturb the equilibrium of consciousness are: ignorance or lack of wisdom, ego, pride of the ego or the sense of 'I', attachment to pleasure, aversion to pain, fear of death and clinging to life (sutra 2.3).

The fluctuations of consciousness created by gross and subtle afflictions are to be silenced through meditation (sutra 2.11).[18]

So meditation is an effective practice for cultivating equanimity and reducing your personal suffering. It not only quiets your mind as you practice, but it also teaches you about how your mind works. As you meditate, you start to become aware of the vrittis and the way your mind gets caught up in them. When you shine that light on them, they lose some of their power over you, and you can start to separate yourself from them.

But not all the vrittis are negative thought patterns. Edwin Bryant defines a vritti as "any sequence of thought, ideas, mental imaging, or cognitive acts performed by the mind, intellect, or ego." In yoga philosophy, any cognitive act interferes with our ability to focus completely on the present and see the world as it truly is. Patanjali states the aim of quieting the mind as follows:

When that is accomplished, the seer abides in its own true nature (sutra 1. 3).[19]

Traditional yogis believe that our souls are divine and therefore our true nature is a state of peace and bliss. But the whirls of consciousness that disturb our minds prevent us from experiencing our true nature. To reach the state of stillness, or samadhi, that allows us to experience the divine within us, we must reach the point where all the whirls of consciousness cease completely. T. K. V. Desikachar has a completely different and very straightforward translation of sutra 1.2, the sutra that defines yoga. In his definition, the moment of quieting the mind through meditation *is* yoga:

Yoga is the ability to direct the mind exclusively toward an object and sustain that direction without any distractions.[20]

Whether the aim of your practice is to experience the divine bliss that is your true nature or simply to become more present and comfortable with uncertainty, quieting the mind is the path that will get you there. As Jill Satterfield says:

Entering into every moment with an open mind might not be totally possible for those of us not yet enlightened, but we can do our best to be lightened in our suffering load. Spiritual maturity then becomes holding less and less, and being open to much, much more.[21]

The Yamas

Lately, Baxter has been focused on cultivating truthfulness in his life. Recently, he was forced to face some hard truths that he'd been hiding even from himself. He finally realized that being overbooked and super busy as a yoga teacher led him to make bad choices that affected him and others close to him in negative ways. He also recognized that despite having told himself that he is not very competitive or motivated by "success," the truth is that he spends energy striving to be "number one" (or at least in the top one hundred) and that this striving was causing him to think and act in ways that were selfish, unhealthy, and limiting. Now he says:

> Starting to see the truth in these areas of my life has opened a door for me to make changes to live with greater *satya* (truthfulness), although the path is often hard and slow. I am now trying to slow my work pace down and set more realistic goals for work where success is defined by deeper personal satisfaction, working with a therapist on improving my emotional openness, and developing new tools for checking in with the truthfulness of my thoughts, statements, and actions and aligning with my higher goals of being of service as a teacher and healer. I am hopeful that these practices will bring me closer and closer to the truth of my life.

According to The Yoga Sutras, *yama*, which means "restraint," is the first branch of yoga. Yamas are yoga's guiding principles for how to conduct yourself in all of your relationships, within your community, and with the world at large. There are five yamas: nonviolence (ahimsa), truthfulness (satya), nonstealing (*asteya*), sexual restraint (*brahmacharya*), and nongreed (*aparigraha*).

There are two different ways you can think about these restraints or "great vows." The first is as a set of rules to follow. From this perspective, adhering to these moral guidelines is as essential for being a yogi as all the other branches of yoga. For example, Gandhi practiced nonviolence through passive resistance in his political work and vegetarianism in his personal life.

Yamas contain essential advice for daily/good living. As they offer a map or guidance that allows us to have enhanced emotional and mental well-being and a more fulfilling and meaningful life, yamas serve as the GPS for our lives. Practicing the yamas leads to greater happiness and spiritual fulfillment not only for the individual but also for those around him/her.

—Ram Rao, "The First Branch of Yoga: The Yamas" from the *Yoga for Healthy Aging* blog

The second is as a set of practices that can help you cultivate equanimity by reducing the conflict in your life and within yourself. As Georg Feuerstein says in *The Deeper Dimensions of Yoga*:

> For as long as we pursue a lifestyle that falls short of these moral virtues, our energies are scattered and we continue to harvest the negative repercussions of our actions.[22]

From this perspective, following these guidelines will reduce the difficulty or even just the drama in your life, which decreases your suffering—as well as that of others—and allows you to experience contentment. Imagine a television soap opera in which everyone stopped harming each other, lying, stealing, cheating on their partners, or taking more than their share. Not much drama in that show!

It's really up to you to decide how best to make use of these guidelines. Of course it can feel overwhelming to try to commit to scrupulously following a challenging set of moral principles. In *Light on Life*, B. K. S. Iyengar recommends that you frame the yamas as "positive" practices that you can cultivate in your life:

> Yama is the cultivation of the positive within us, not merely a suppression of what we consider to be its diabolical opposite. If we consider the nonpractice of yama in this way, we will be doomed, not to encourage the good, but to ricochet between extremes of vice and virtue, which will cause us nothing but pain and which have no beneficial effect on the world. Cultivate the positive, abjure the negative. Little by little, one will arrive.[23]

Nonviolence (Ahimsa)

Ahimsa is considered the "fundamental" yama. It includes nonviolence in thought as well as action and covers your relationship to all living things. The negative consequences of violent acts are clear in current events and history as well as our personal stories. Over and over we observe one act of violence leading to another and then another. So practicing nonviolence in your life helps foster both your own inner peace and peace in your community.

Ahimsa also means "nonharming" so it includes refraining from actions or thoughts that harm another, whether physically, mentally, or emotionally. Practicing nonharming also means refraining from harming yourself, as illustrated by Evelyn's story in the introduction of this chapter, and choosing the appropriate yoga practices for your particular phase in life. From a positive perspective, practicing nonviolence means cultivating compassion for others and kindness toward yourself.

Truthfulness (Satya)

Truthfulness includes practicing honesty in action, speech, and thought. Lying or misleading others is a form of harm because it violates the trust others have in us. So many of the conflicts between us, including violence, are the result of keeping secrets and then telling lies to cover them up. So, like practicing nonviolence, practicing truthfulness helps foster inner peace and reduces conflicts in your relationships. However, because ahimsa is the fundamental yama, you always need to consider nonharming when you practice truthfulness. Use compassion when you speak and aim to cause the least harm possible, even remaining silent if necessary.

The word *satya* also means "real," "genuine," "honest," and "virtuous." One meaning of being "real" is that you see the true nature of reality and that you communicate it honestly, rather than clinging to how you wish the world would be or telling people what they want to hear.

In addition to your conduct with others, practicing truthfulness includes being honest with—and not lying to—yourself. Baxter's story of his personal practice of truthfulness illustrates this perfectly, and our story about Nancy at the beginning of the book illustrates the importance of being honest with yourself about your changing abilities and needs as you age.

Nonstealing (Asteya)

Stealing, of course, means taking things that belong to others, including both material things and ideas (such as taking credit for someone else's work). Of course, stealing is not just wrong on its own; it is a form of harming as well. It violates the person you steal from and leads to other types of harm, including lies, violence, betrayal, and so on, in the attempt to cover up the original crime.

The word *asteya* also means "noncoveting" and "nondesire." Even if you don't commit crimes to obtain the objects of your desire, coveting material goods can cause you to overspend, even go into debt, which is not only stressful for you but can ruin your family. Or maybe the desire for material possessions or even just "success" simply means you work at a stressful, unsatisfying job. In general, being in a state of desire for what you don't have creates a cycle of dissatisfaction because what you have is never enough, and you're always looking to acquire more. Naturally all of these forms of coveting are impediments to your peace of mind.

Practicing asteya means cultivating contentment with what you have and what you don't have (see "Contentment" on page 200) and letting go of these desires.

Sexual Restraint (Brahmacharya)

Sexual restraint is a complex topic for our culture. The original meaning of *brahmacharya* in The Yoga Sutras is "chastity," which means refraining from sex completely. That's because the yogic path described in The Yoga Sutras was intended for practitioners who were unmarried and lived apart from the rest of society. In modern times, we ordinary "householders" consider brahmacharya to be sexual responsibility. For example, B. K. S. Iyengar says that for him, practicing brahmacharya meant being faithful to his wife.

Not practicing sexual restraint is a form of harming. If you are reckless in your sexual conduct, well, we're back to the soap opera territory with lies, jealousy, pain, and even violence. Of course, these days we understand the damage that is caused by sexual abuse in all its forms, whether that means sexual harassment or predatory behavior by those in power. But exactly how you interpret sexual responsibility depends on your personal commitments, your religion if you practice one, and the culture in which you live.

Nongreed (Aparigraha)

Nongreed means limiting your possessions to what is truly necessary and living a life of voluntary simplicity. In yoga philosophy, having too many possessions is considered an "indulgence" that distracts you from spiritual development. Anyone who has known someone who hoards (a behavior that tends to become more problematic with age) understands how having too many possessions sucks up time and energy and creates fear and anxiety at the thought of losing what has been accumulated. From a positive perspective, practicing aparigraha means cultivating an attitude of generosity toward others and being willing to share both your resources and your time.

The word *aparigraha* also means "nonpossessiveness," "nonholding," "nonindulgence," and "nonacquisitiveness." An important aspect of nonholding includes not clinging to ideas or emotions. Sometimes these are negative emotions, such as fear, worry, anxiety, grief, anger, rage, and jealousy, which cloud your judgment and disturb your equanimity. Practicing aparigraha means letting go of negative emotions rather than allowing them to become obsessions.

At other times we hold onto ideas that give us a sense of security, such as the lives we plan for ourselves or the images we have of who we are. When circumstances change, clinging to these beliefs prevents you from living in the present. For example, maybe a marriage you once thought would last forever ends in a divorce or years of striving for success in a certain job or profession ends in failure or someone important to you dies unexpectedly. Or maybe you've always been the strong one but now you need to turn to others for help. Practicing aparigraha means letting go of what once gave you a sense of security and opening up to new opportunities and paths that will take you forward.

CONTENTMENT

At thirty-seven, our colleague Elizabeth Ann Gibbs, a middle-class, African-American woman, who was divorced, a single parent with a full-time job in broadcasting, and studying for a Master's degree in communications, felt that she had to "do it all," be a "credit to the race," and prove herself competent, capable, connected, and "enough." But inside she felt crazy:

> Underneath my struggling and juggling, I was constipated and stressed. I developed TMJ (temporal mandibular joint dysfunction). There was not enough time, not enough energy, and not enough of me to go around and do all that was expected of me and all that I expected from myself.[24]

It was then that she turned to yoga. Practicing the poses helped her manage her stress, but she also felt that yoga was doing something else. When she finally started reading through The Yoga Sutras, she was immediately drawn to sutra 2.42 and this quote from I. K. Taimni:

> It is necessary for the aspirant for the Yogic life to cultivate contentment of the highest order because without it there is no possibility of keeping the mind in a condition of equilibrium.[25]

Beth says that she immediately recognized that contentment was a concept that "resonated deeply to my feelings of not being enough." Later on, when she was at a yoga retreat, away from home and family and work, she found herself "floating somewhere between here and there at the same time," experiencing grace, surrender, and contentment.

In our materialistic and success-oriented culture, we are bombarded with messages telling us we need to do more, buy more, and be more.

For the pleasures that come from the world bear in them sorrows to come. They come and they go, they are transient: not in them do the wise find joy.

But he who on this earth, before his departure, can endure the storms of desire and wrath, this man is a Yogi, this man has joy.

He has inner joy, he has inner gladness, and he has found inner Light.

— Juan Mascaró, translator, *The Bhagavad Gita*

So we become caught up in an endless cycle of desire and dissatisfaction, which benefits the economy but not necessarily our equanimity. For us, the concept of contentment is the antidote. Here's another definition of contentment from T. K. V. Desikachar:

> Contentment, or the ability to be comfortable with what we have and what we do not have.[26]

To us, this means that there are many unpleasant situations in your life that you cannot change, some minor (traffic jams, lost items) and some major (death, divorce, loss of a job). In these circumstances, when you normally would react with anger, anxiety, envy, frustration, or sorrow, you might be able to choose to react instead with contentment.

The term "contentment" in this context can be confusing to people. Students ask, "How can I be content when something bad happens?" Someone struggling with depression will ask, "How can I just tell myself to be happy?" So we suggest using different language, such as "I can be okay with this." Nina Rook says that her yoga practice helped support her after the early death of her beloved elder sister with whom she had planned to spend her future. When she was feeling "unmoored" with no clear path forward, yoga allowed her to feel comfortable with uncertainty, without the anxiety the situation would have triggered earlier in her life, before yoga.

In addition, there are many people who feel they can't be content until something positive happens to make their lives complete. Maybe that means something material, like owning your own home, or maybe it's a change in life status, like getting married or achieving career success. Being content with what you have and what you don't have means letting go of the illusion that you need to complete some kind of life list to achieve happiness. After ten years of trying to get pregnant, Leza Lowitz turned to her meditation practice to help her come to terms with her infertility. She says she practiced to help get herself outside of her own "story" and "suffering," and that little by little her own life became "happier and somehow free."

Mindfulness practices, including meditation, breath practices, and asanas, can be helpful for cultivating contentment because they anchor you in the present moment, preventing you from focusing on regrets about the past or worries about the future. Meditation practices that specifically focus on gratitude or compassion for others can be especially effective. You can also use the technique of cultivating the opposite we described under "Practice" above. This technique will also help you cultivate contentment in your relationships. Sutra 1.33 in The Yoga Sutras, translated by Swami Jnaneshvara, describes it this way:

> In relationships, the mind becomes purified by cultivating feelings of friendliness toward those who are happy, compassion for those who are suffering, goodwill toward those who are virtuous, and indifference or neutrality toward those we perceive as wicked or evil.[27]

Cultivating contentment is not only necessary for equanimity, as it helps prevent negative emotions that disturb your peace of mind, but according to The Yoga Sutras, it is also necessary for happiness. Edwin Bryant says that this form of happiness is "inherent in the mind when it is tranquil and content."

Beth says that the ability to be present and be content with all the joys and problems of her life is what finally led her to experience the feeling of being enough:

> I rejoice in the fact that underneath the "African," underneath the "American," and underneath the "woman," is a being who can occasionally and surprisingly "be here now" and be content. In those moments, I can rest amid chaos and be present in the midst of my life with all its joys and problems. I can experience this and me at the same time. I am competent, capable, connected, and a credit to universal consciousness in all its forms.[28]

THERE ARE MANY PATHS

Here in the West, even though most of us who practice yoga are householders (as opposed to monks) and very few of us are dedicating our lives to the contemplative aspects of yoga, there has been a tendency to identify the path described in The Yoga Sutras as the *only* path. In fact, the eight-fold path that The Yoga Sutras describes is Raja Yoga, the path of concentration and meditation with the aim of achieving samadhi (spiritual absorption).

On the other hand, in the Bhagavad Gita, which preceded The Yoga Sutras by approximately 800 years, Arjuna is a householder and man of action, and the yoga that Krishna is encouraging him to practice is "karma yoga," the yoga of work. This is the path of selfless service, in which every action becomes a "sacrifice," where you surrender the outcome of your

Yoga is like an ancient river with countless rapids, eddies, loops, tributaries, and backwaters, extending over a vast, colourful terrain of many different habitats. So, when we speak of Yoga, we speak of a multitude of paths and orientations with contrasting theoretical frameworks and occasionally incompatible goals.

—Georg Feuerstein, *Yoga Journal*, March/April 1990

action to the divine. This is the path taken by Mohandas K. Gandhi, who lived a life dedicated to social activism, and it is also the path that inspires our colleague Ram Rao, who commits much of his free time to selfless service.

Even though Krishna recommends the yoga of work for Arjuna, he tells Arjuna that there is more than one path. *The Bhagavad Gita* states:

> Some by the Yoga of meditation, and by the grace of the Spirit, see the Spirit in themselves; some by the Yoga of the vision of Truth; and others by the Yoga of work (sutra 13.24).[29]

Yoga has been evolving dramatically since then. In his book, *The Yoga Tradition*, Georg Feuerstein identified six different paths associated with Hinduism alone, and there are also "yogas" within Jainism, Buddhism, and Sikhism. At this point, we've lost count of all the paths there are!

The takeaway is this: there is no single path, and you should find the path that works for you. The particular path you take can depend on many things, including your natural disposition, your religious background, your particular phase in life, and a teacher or community that you resonate with.

Now some of you may be wondering: "Which of these paths am I on?" "Do I have to follow one path, or even any path at all?" "Does it matter if I mix it up?"

We like Feuerstein's perspective on these questions in *The Yoga Tradition*:

> In our struggle for self-understanding and psycho-spiritual growth, we can benefit immensely from a liberal exposure to India's spiritual legacy. We need not, of course, become converts to any path, or accept yogic ideas and practices without questioning. C. G. Jung's warning that we should not attempt to transplant Eastern teachings into the West rings true at a certain level; mere imitation definitely does more harm than good. The reason is that if we adopt ideas and lifestyles without truly assimilating them emotionally and intellectually, we run the risk of living inauthentic lives.[30]

When Baxter originally started studying yoga in the early nineties, all of his teachers were from the Iyengar lineage. That path provided him with a good understanding of physical and energetic alignment, as well as mental focus and discipline. Then in 2001, inspired by the teachings of T. K. V. Desikachar, he began to study *viniyoga* and the work of

Krishnamacharya, focusing particularly on the tradition of working individually with students. In the past few years, he has been drawn to the writings of Pandit Rajmani Tigunait, the head of the Himalayan Institute. He says this shifting path feels organic and natural, and it has changed the way he both practices and teaches for the better.

So don't get attached to one path or to one teacher's interpretations of what yoga means just because it's the one you started out with. Try to keep an open mind and, if you haven't already, start to learn as much as you can about yoga philosophy and the history of yoga. As you learn about different paths and concepts, you may be surprised to find many more ideas and practices that are helpful for you. This is the end of our exploration of yoga philosophy, but we hope it's the beginning of a lifelong journey for you.

PART TWO

ESSENTIAL YOGA POSES AND VINYASAS

THIS SECTION PROVIDES PHOTOGRAPHS OF AND INSTRUCTIONS on how to practice all four versions of the poses we've included in this book. The poses are listed in alphabetical order by English name (the names we use throughout the book), with the traditional Sanskrit name in parentheses. Due to space constraints, we're only able to include very basic information about the poses. If you're interested in learning more about alignment in yoga poses, ask your favorite yoga teacher.

Remember, if you're new to the practice or recovering from an illness or injury, it's always best to start with the easiest version of the pose and gradually work up to the most challenging one (if that is accessible to you). If you're having trouble with balance, try practicing your standing poses near a wall so you can reach for it if needed. For everyone, if the instructions say to do something you're not comfortable with, feel free to do what's best for you!

Symmetrical poses—Some of these poses are symmetrical, which means that the right sides and left sides of your body look the same while you're in the pose. Examples are Downward-Facing Dog Pose, Cobra Pose, and Standing Forward Bend. In this case, you can either do the pose once or repeat if desired.

Asymmetrical poses—Other poses are asymmetrical poses, which means that the right and left sides of your body look different from each other while you're in the pose. Examples are Triangle Pose, Easy Sitting Twist, and Reclined Leg Stretch. For these poses, we provide information on how to practice the pose on the right side only. After completing the right side, you should always repeat the pose on left side. Repeating an asymmetrical pose means doing it once on each side and then repeating it a second time on each side.

Dynamic poses and flow sequences—Photographic illustrations of all the dynamic poses and flow sequences that appear in the book are presented at the end of this part. These illustrate the step-by-step movements you should take with each inhalation and exhalation. Like static poses, some of these dynamic poses and flow sequences are symmetrical and some are asymmetrical. For asymmetrical dynamic poses and flow sequences, doing the sequence "once" means doing it once on each side.

Prescriptions — For each pose in this chapter, we list some of the applications for the pose that we feel are particularly beneficial. But these are just some highlights. As you explore the poses on your own or learn more about them from other teachers, you may find many additional uses for them.

Happy practicing!

ARMS OVERHEAD POSE (*Urdhva Hastasana*)

This simple, energizing pose provides the postural benefits of Mountain Pose while stretching and strengthening your arms and shoulders and opening your chest. We prescribe this pose for lower back pain, upper back stiffness, posture, fatigue, and arthritis of the shoulders and arms.

CAUTIONS: If you have a shoulder injury or pain, take your arms up slowly, only going as far as you can without pain. If any version causes lower back pain, take your arms only partway up or side bend in version 4 only to a pain-free distance. Those with newly diagnosed or poorly controlled high blood pressure should only hold for the pose for four breaths.

Version 1: Classic Pose

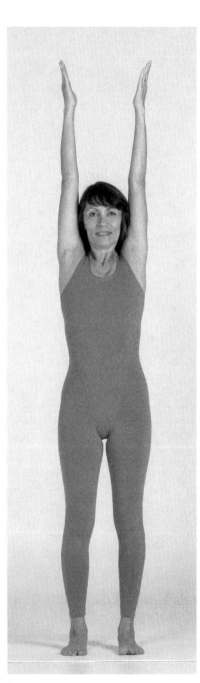

Start in Mountain Pose with straight arms. Lift your arms forward and up alongside your ears, with palms facing each other. If you can't keep your arms straight, take them wider apart. Keep your legs strong and lengthen upward through your spine to the crown of your head as if growing taller, encouraging a slight, even arch of your spine. Lengthen up through the sides of your body, from your hips all the way through your fingertips. Relax the sides of your neck as you lift your outer shoulder blades. If you notice that your back is arching deeply or your front lower ribs are jutting forward, relax your front lower ribs toward your spine, even if your arms release a bit forward. To come out, lower your arms and return to Mountain Pose.

Version 2: Block between Hands

This option builds more upper back, shoulder, and arm strength than the classic pose.

From Mountain Pose, take the block between your hands, press your palms against the small ends of the block, and straighten your arms. Lift your arms forward and up alongside your ears as you press your palms into the block. Then follow the alignment instructions for the classic pose. In this version you may not be able to bring your straight arms up as high, so stop when you feel your elbows bend. Because holding the block takes extra effort, start with shorter holds and gradually work up to longer holds over time.

To come out, press your hands into the block as you lower your arms.

Version 3: Bound Hands

This option increases shoulder flexibility while stretching the muscles of forearms, wrists, and hands.

In Mountain Pose, interlace your fingers and turn your palms down toward the floor. Keeping your fingers interlaced, pull your wrists apart. Raise your arms overhead, as far as they will go with straight elbows. If your hands are in the correct position, your palms will be facing the ceiling when your arms are overhead. Then follow the alignment instructions for the classic pose.

To come out, lower your arms and then release your hands and shake them out. Optionally, repeat with your fingers interlaced the opposite way.

Version 4: Crescent Moon

This option provides a full side stretch from your hips up through your hands, releasing tension in both muscles and fascia while building core strength.

Start in the classic pose. Then simultaneously lengthen and side bend your torso and arms a few inches over to your right side until you feel a moderate stretch on the left side of your body. Keep your hips and chest facing forward and either look forward or turn your head down to look at your right foot. Keep your arms and legs energized and strong, as you firm your right side and relax your left side.

To come out, maintain strong legs as you lift back up to the classic pose. Then repeat on the left side.

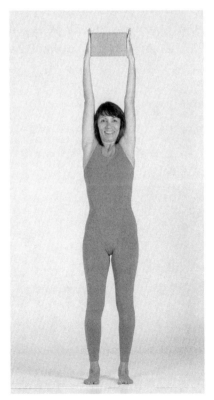
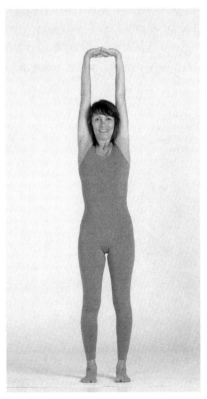
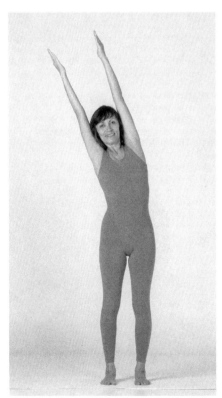

2   3   4

BOAT POSE (*Navasana*)

This energizing and challenging pose strengthens the muscles at the front of your body, especially your upper leg muscles and the core muscles of your abdomen, and improves balance. We prescribe this pose for core strength, concentration, and cultivating equanimity.

CAUTIONS: Those with abdominal hernias or women with abdominal wall separation need to be cautious in this pose, so it does not worsen the herniation. Try firming your belly toward your spine and holding the pose for just a few breaths. Those with lower back pain should start with version 2 or skip the pose altogether if it worsens symptoms. Those with newly diagnosed or poorly controlled high blood pressure should hold the pose for only four breaths.

Version 1: Classic Pose (*Paripurna Navasana*)

Sit with your knees bent and your feet on the floor, and hold the backs of your knees. Step your feet a bit closer to your hips and lean your chest back. Keeping your head and neck over your shoulders, lean back until your feet come off the floor and you find your balance spot. Straighten your knees and angle your legs upward and forward, with your toes around eye level. Keep your spine long and strong while slightly rounding it, and lift your arms alongside your legs, parallel with the floor.

To come out, bend your knees and return your feet to the floor, as you bring your chest and head upright. Sit for a moment in Easy Sitting Pose or with legs straight out in front of you.

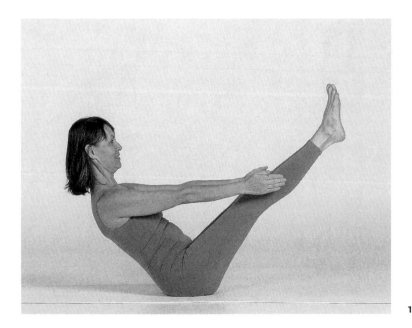

1

Version 2: Knees Bent, Hands on the Floor

This alternative is for beginners, those with general weakness, those with back problems, or those with balance problems.

Start with your knees bent and feet on the floor as in the classic pose but place your hands on the floor alongside your hips. Now walk your hands about one foot behind you, bending your elbows backward a bit, and lean your torso back about 30–45 degrees, head balanced over your shoulders. Swing your shins up to be parallel with the floor, keeping your legs either together or just slightly apart.

To come out, bend your knees and return your feet to the floor while walking your hands forward and bringing your chest to a vertical position. Shake out your hands and wrists.

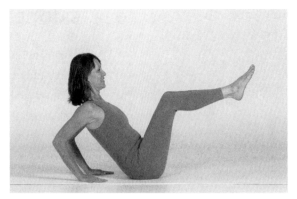

2

Version 3: Knees Bent, Hands off the Floor

This alternative is for those who find the classic version too challenging and version 2 too easy.

Come into the classic pose, lifting your shins to be parallel with the floor instead of straightening your legs. Once you are balanced, release your hands from the backs of your legs and reach your arms forward, parallel with the floor. The angle between chest and thighs can be from 90–110 degrees.

To come out, use the steps for the classic pose.

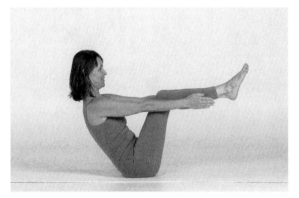

3

Version 4: Half Boat Pose (*Arda Navasana*)

This is a more challenging option for your core muscles that is easier to balance in than the classic pose.

Come into the classic pose or version 3. Mindfully lower your chest and legs at the same time, keeping your chin tucked a bit toward your chest, until shoulders and heels are about a foot off the floor and toes are at eye level. As you lower down, allow the back of your pelvis and your lower back to round to the floor, so more of your back body is resting on the floor than in the other versions.

To come out, lower your chest, head, and legs down to the floor.

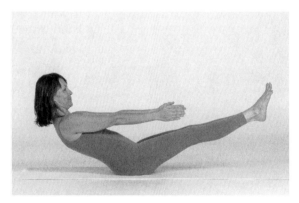

4

BRIDGE POSE (*Setu Bandha Sarvangasana*)

This accessible, mildly energizing backbend allows you to mobilize your spine and open your chest, while at the same time strengthening your legs, back, and shoulders. We prescribe this pose for lower back pain, spinal bone strength, circulation, improving breath capacity, depression, stress, quieting the mind, and as a counter pose for forward bends and twists.

CAUTIONS: Never roll your head side to side in the pose, as this can injure your neck. Those with neck pain should come into the pose slowly and stop lifting if pain occurs, or skip the pose entirely. If the pose worsens back pain, skip it. If you experience knee pain in the classic version, try placing a block between your knees and squeeze the block while practicing. If that doesn't help, do any other version instead.

Version 1: Classic Pose

Start in version 4 of Relaxation Pose, with heels about four inches from hips. With thighs parallel, push down into your feet and lift your hips straight up, maintaining your natural lower back arch. Stop when the stretch on your front body is strong or your knees come apart. Press the backs of your upper arms firmly down while actively lifting the lower tip of your breastbone. Now, either keep pressing your arms firmly down into the floor or roll your upper arm bones under your chest and clasp your hands together under your body. Keep your head and neck relaxed and centered.

To come out, move your arms out to your sides, then lower your hips straight down to the floor.

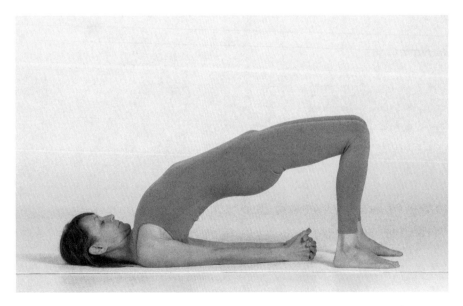

1

Version 2: Supported with Low/Medium Block

This is an option for a restorative experience that still provides the benefits of a backbend.

With a block near your hip, follow the steps for coming into the classic pose. As you enter the backbend, lift your hips just high enough to slip the block crosswise on its medium or lowest height under the top part of your buttocks, just below your waist. Rest your pelvis fully on the block. Press your feet down just enough to keep your legs parallel with each other and lift the lower tip of your breastbone as in the classic pose. Take either arm position from the classic pose.

To come out, press into your feet, lift your hips off the block, and slide the block out of the way. Then lower your hips gently to the floor.

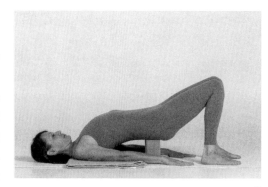

2

Version 3: Supported with High Block

This is a supported option that provides more stretch to the front of your hips, abdomen, and chest. If this version causes pain in your lower back or neck, practice version 2.

Use the steps for version 2, but as you lift your hips up, come onto the balls of your feet so you can slip the block crosswise under your pelvis on its highest height. As you lower your pelvis onto the block, your heels should be able to come to the floor. If they don't, come out and turn the block down to a lower height. Press your feet down just enough to keep your legs parallel with each other and lift the lower tip of your breastbone as in the classic pose. Take either arm position from the classic pose.

To come out, use the steps for version 2, lifting your hips if necessary.

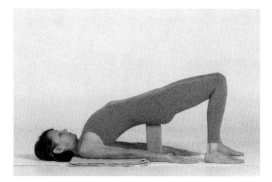

3

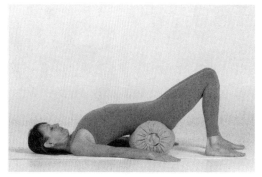

4

Version 4: Supported with Bolster

This is an option for a restorative experience and an alternative for those with a sensitive lower back or pelvis.

To come into the pose, follow the steps for version 2, using a bolster instead of a block. When you slide the bolster crosswise under your pelvis and release down onto it, make sure the entire bolster is supporting the back of your pelvis (not your lower back).

To come out, use the steps for the classic pose.

CAT-COW POSE, DYNAMIC (*Cakravakasana*)

This gentle, dynamic pose slowly warms up your spine as it strengthens your arms, shoulders, and the bones of your spine and wrists. We prescribe this pose for lower back pain, stress, fatigue, circulation issues, stiffness and arthritis of the hips and spine, spine health, improving breath capacity, and depression.

CAUTIONS: If you have wrist pain, try coming onto your fingertips, making fists, or coming onto your forearms instead (with shoulders over elbows). If you have lower back pain, modify the amount of arch or rounding so you don't experience pain as you move.

Version 1: Starting Position

This is the neutral hands and knees position you take before moving in and out of Dynamic Cat-Cow Pose and that you return to after you've completed your rounds.

Place a folded blanket crosswise in the middle of your mat. Then come into a hands and knees position, with your knees, shins, and tops of your feet on the blanket, your hands on the mat, your hips directly over your knees, and your shoulders directly above your wrists. Spread your fingers and firmly press your hands into the mat as you firm the muscles around your elbows to keep your arms straight. With your spine parallel to the floor, lengthen from your tailbone to the crown of your head.

After completing your set of Dynamic Cat-Cow Pose, sit back on your heels and shake out your wrists.

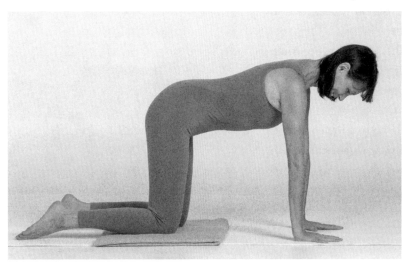

1

Version 2: Cow Pose

This is the first position in the Dynamic Cat-Cow Pose sequence, which takes your spine into a backbend shape, from your tailbone to the crown of your head. This strengthens your back muscles while stretching the front of your belly and chest, encouraging a full inhalation.

To come into the pose, as you start your inhalation, gradually arch your spine into a backbend by moving from your pelvis. Lift your tailbone and sitting bones up as your pelvis tips forward over your leg bones, relax your belly, and lift your chest and head forward. Keep your collarbones broad as you continue pressing your hands into the floor and firming the muscles around your elbows.

When you're ready to exhale, you'll move into Cat Pose.

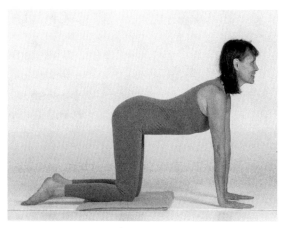

2

Version 3: Cat Pose

This is the second position in the Dynamic Cat-Cow Pose sequence, which takes your spine into a forward rounding position. This strengthens your abdominal and front chest muscles, while stretching your back muscles.

To come into the pose, as you start your exhalation from Cow Pose, gradually round your spine toward the ceiling by moving from your pelvis. Turn your tailbone and sitting bones down as your pelvis tips backward, hollow your belly toward your spine, and release your neck and head toward the floor. Keep your neck relaxed as you continue pressing your hands into the floor and firming the muscles around your elbows.

When you're ready to inhale, you'll move back into Cow Pose. If you've finished your final round, inhale and return to the starting position.

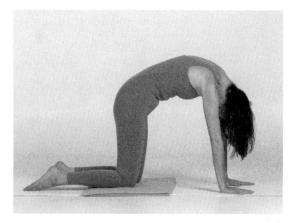

3

Version 4: Sitting on a Chair

This is an alternative for those who cannot bear weight on their arms or cannot get down to the floor.

Place a chair with a firm seat on your mat. Sit near the front edge of the chair, with both feet on the ground, your thighs parallel to each other, and your knees directly over your heels. Straighten your arms and rest your hands on your thighs or knees. Create an inner lift of your spine from your sitting bones to the crown of your head.

To come into the Cow position, on an inhalation, gradually rock your pelvis forward as you lift and arch your spine into a gentle backbend. Allow your chest to move forward and up and lift your chin a few inches. To come into the Cat position, on an exhalation, gradually rock your pelvis back as you round your spine gently toward the back of your chair. Drop your chin a few inches toward your chest.

When you've finished your final round, return to the starting position.

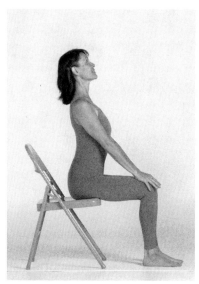

4

CHILD'S POSE (*Balasana*)

This restful, quieting pose stretches your lower back and the fronts of your ankles and feet. We prescribe this pose for lower back pain, stress, anxiety, insomnia, quieting the mind, as a counter pose for backbends and twists, and as a resting pose between other floor poses.

CAUTIONS: Those with knee, hip, or ankle pain, try version 3 or 4. If you still feel pain, skip the pose. Although many people with lower back pain find this pose helpful, avoid the pose if it worsens your pain. Those with neck pain should be careful with the placement of your neck and head to avoid worsening symptoms.

Version 1: Classic Pose

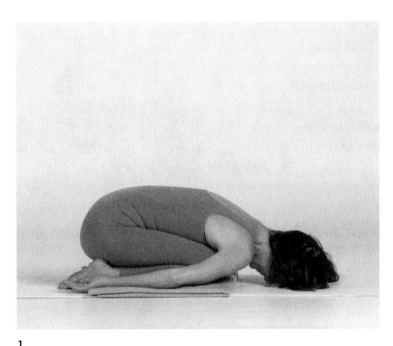

1

Place a thin blanket on your mat and come into a hands and knees position on the blanket. Keeping knees about hip-distance apart, slide your feet closer together so your big toes touch. Slowly lower your hips back and down toward your heels. Gently round your back forward and down, with your chest toward or onto your thighs. Release your head, resting your forehead on the floor. Sweep your arms back alongside your body, with the backs of your hands near your feet. Release your shoulder blades away from your spine.

To come out, place your palms next to your knees and use your arms to help you roll up and sit back on your heels.

Version 2: Arms Forward Version

This is an option for opening your chest and upper back and a good preparation for Arms Overhead Pose or backbends.

Come into the classic pose, stretching your arms as far forward as you can. With your arms parallel and elbows straight, press your hands into the floor. After thirty seconds in this active position, relax your elbows to the floor, decreasing the stretch of your arms. This relaxed arm version may even feel more restorative than having your hands by your feet.

To come out, follow the steps for the classic pose.

Version 3: Support for Knees or Ankles

This is an alternative for those with tight ankles or knee joints. CAUTION: Never use a roll behind your knees if you've had an anterior cruciate ligament (ACL) tear or repair.

If only your ankles are tight, roll a blanket or towel into a two- to three-inch roll and place it under your ankle joints before you take Child's Pose. If your knees are tight, arthritic, or painful when bent, place the roll behind both knees when you are in hands and knees position. Then slowly lower your hips back and down as in the classic pose. When your thighs reach the support, ensure that both knees feel good. If you have problems in both your ankles and your knees, use both supports.

To come out, use the steps for the classic pose, removing the props only after you return to hands and knees position.

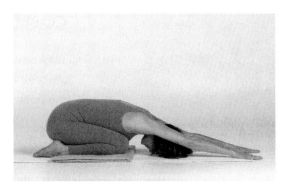

2

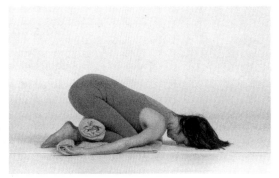

3

Version 4: Restorative Alternative

This option provides a restorative experience and is an alternative for those with tight or painful hips, knees, or ankles.

Position a bolster lengthwise in front of you. After you lower your hips toward your heels, widen your knees about two feet apart and slide the end of your bolster toward your hips, up against your lower belly but not under your hips. Then lower your belly, chest, and head onto the bolster, turning your head to one side as you release your buttocks toward your heels. Make sure your entire front belly and chest are supported; if not, try adding more props. Midway through the pose, turn your head in the opposite direction.

To come out, use your hands to slowly roll up to sitting.

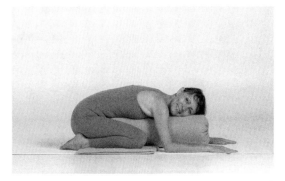

4

COBBLER'S POSE (*Baddha Konasana*)

This quieting seated pose stretches your inner thighs and improves the range of motion of your hip joints while strengthening your back muscles. We prescribe this pose for posture, spine health, stress, quieting the mind, and as preparation for other seated and standing poses.

CAUTIONS: Those with lower back pain, herniated discs, or sacroiliac problems, use caution when entering version 4 or skip it entirely. Those with osteoporosis should skip version 4. Those with knee pain may need to keep their feet farther forward to open up the knee joints.

Version 1: Classic Pose

Start in Easy Sitting Pose. Move your knees apart until you can bring the soles of your feet together at about twelve to eighteen inches from your hips, with baby toes resting on the floor. Press the soles of your feet together or let the inner edges of your feet drop open. If your knees don't drop below the level of your waist, try version 2. Rest your hands on your knees or hold your ankles or feet, whichever is more comfortable. Create an internal lift from your sitting bones through your spine and up to the crown of your head, while maintaining the natural curves of your spine.

To come out, use your hands to bring your bent knees up to center, then lengthen your legs out in front of you.

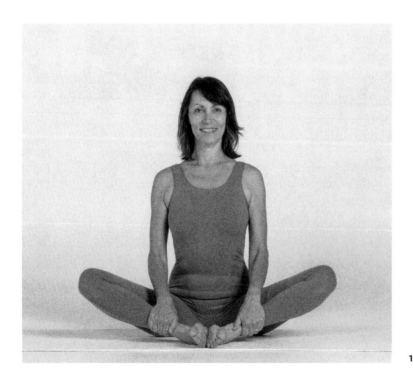

1

Version 2: Propping Hips and/or Knees

This is an alternative for those who can't sit comfortably in the classic pose and those whose knees are too high in that version.

Choose a prop to sit on that allows you to maintain good posture with less effort and that releases tension in your hips, allowing your knees to release toward the ground. Sit on the edge of the prop and follow the steps for coming into the classic pose. Support your knees with props that are high enough to allow them to rest easily. If you have only one side that rides high, prop both knees so they are even.

To come out, move your knee supports to the sides and then use the steps for the classic pose.

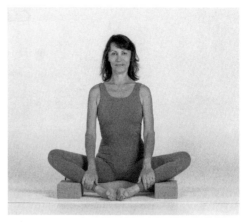

3

Version 3: Back Support

This is an alternative for those who have trouble maintaining good posture or who tire quickly. It's also an option for a meditation or breath practice position.

Feel free to use props as in version 2. Come to Easy Sitting Pose with your back near a wall. Then scoot your buttocks as close to the wall as you can, leaning slightly forward from your hips. Roll your spine up to touch the wall and bring your legs into Cobbler's Pose. Ideally, the back of your pelvis and shoulder blades rest against the wall, your lower back is slightly off the wall, and your head is positioned above your shoulders.

To come out, use the steps for the classic pose.

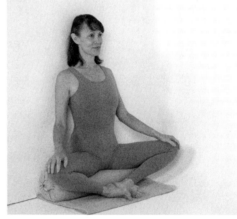

2

Version 4: Cobbler's Forward Bend

This option provides more stretch in your hip joints and your spinal muscles.

Come into version 1, 2, or 3, holding your ankles or feet. Fold forward, initially tipping from your hips until your pelvis stops rolling forward. Then gently round forward without pulling your spine down with your arms. Once you feel stretching sensations around your hips, buttocks, hamstrings, and/or lower back, do not bend any farther. If you experience knee or back pain in the pose, come out immediately.

To come out, lift up to vertical and then use the steps for the classic pose.

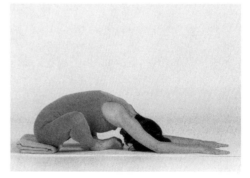

4

COBRA POSE (*Bhujangasana*)

This active, energizing backbend strengthens your upper, middle, and lower back, from your pelvis to the back of your head, while stretching the front of your body from front hips to chin. Versions 1, 3, and 4 also strengthen and stabilize your shoulder joints and shoulder blades. We prescribe this pose for posture, spine health, fatigue, and depression.

CAUTIONS: Those with lower back pain in the pose should firm your belly toward your spine. If the pose worsens back or neck pain, try Supported Backbend instead. Those with abdominal hernias or women with abdominal wall separation should practice this pose with care so it does not worsen your condition, or try Bridge Pose instead. If you have wrist or hand pain, try version 3 or 4 of Cobra Pose or any version of Locust Pose.

Version 1: Classic Pose

Lie on your belly, with your chin or forehead on the floor and the tops of your feet turned down, with toes pointing back. Bend your elbows and place your hands palms down—fingers pointing forward—by the sides of your rib cage (the exact position depends on your body type). Press your palms down and slowly roll up until your arms are straight and your shoulders are over your wrists, with your legs lengthening along the floor. Move your shoulder blades down, firming them against your back, and widen your collarbones. If you can't straighten your arms while keeping your legs on the floor, keep your arms slightly bent.

To come out, bend your elbows and lower down to the starting position.

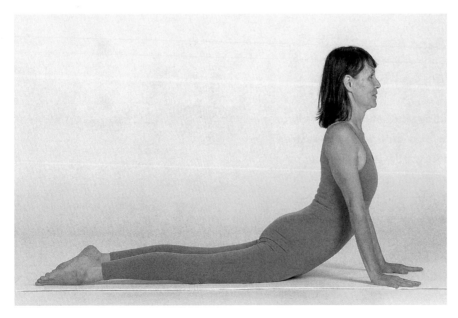

1

Version 2: Low Cobra Pose

This is an alternative for those with stiff spines or wrist pain. It's also an option for increasing upper back strength.

Take the starting position for the classic pose, hands in line with your shoulders. Press lightly into your hands and roll up about six inches off the floor. Use your back muscles to maintain this lower position, with elbows bent and arms parallel to the sides of your body, hands still light on the floor. Lift your head in line with the arch of the backbend, not farther back. Work with your shoulder blades and collarbones as for the classic pose.

To come out, use the steps for the classic pose.

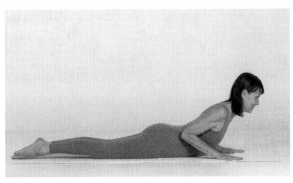

2

Version 3: Sphinx Pose

This is an alternative for those with stiff spines, general weakness, or wrist problems.

Take the starting position for the classic pose, with hands in line with your shoulders. Press into your hands and roll up about six inches off the floor. As you come up, with your forearms parallel, slide your hands and forearms forward until your elbows are under your shoulder joints. Press your forearms down while lifting your chest up, moving your shoulder blades down, widening your collarbones, and bringing your head to a neutral position over your shoulders.

To come out, slide your elbows out to the sides as you lower your chest and head down to the floor. Then follow the steps for the classic pose.

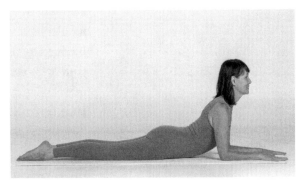

3

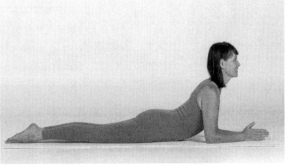

4

Version 4: Sphinx with Palms Together

This alternative is an easier version of Sphinx Pose, which is especially helpful for those with shoulder problems.

Follow the steps for version 3, but instead of keeping your forearms parallel, bring your palms together. Press your forearms down while lifting your chest up, moving your shoulder blades down, widening your collarbones, and bringing your head to a neutral position over your shoulders.

To come out, use the steps for version 3.

DOWNWARD-FACING DOG POSE
(*Adho Mukha Svanasana*)

This versatile, all-over stretching and strengthening pose opens your shoulders and upper back, stretches and lengthens the muscles in your lower back and the backs of your hips and legs, and builds strength in your upper body, front thighs, and core abdominal muscles. We prescribe this pose for lower back pain, spine health, stress, bone strength for hips and wrists, circulation issues, improving breath capacity, and anxiety.

CAUTIONS: Those with lower back pain should try version 2 or 3. Those with wrist or hand pain should practice version 3 or 4. Those with nasal congestion or sinus pressure should practice Half Downward-Facing Dog Pose instead. If you have a shoulder injury or pain, straighten your arms carefully, only going as far as you can without pain. Those with newly diagnosed or poorly controlled high blood pressure should practice Half Downward-Facing Dog Pose instead, or hold the full pose for only four breaths.

Version 1: Classic Pose

From a hands and knees position, move your hands forward about one hand length and turn your toes under. Press your hands firmly into the floor and straighten your elbows. Lift your knees off the floor and push your hips up and back, away from your hands, as you gradually begin to straighten your legs. Release your heels onto or toward the floor and lengthen from your wrists to your sitting bones. Keep some muscular tone in your belly if you tend to sway your back, and float your head in line with your spine.

To come out, bend your knees and bring them lightly to the floor.

Version 2: Bent Knees

This is an alternative for those with tight hamstrings, calves, hips, or lower back muscles that cause your lower back to round when your legs are straight. It's also a good alternative for those with back pain.

To practice this version, rather than straightening your legs, bend your knees

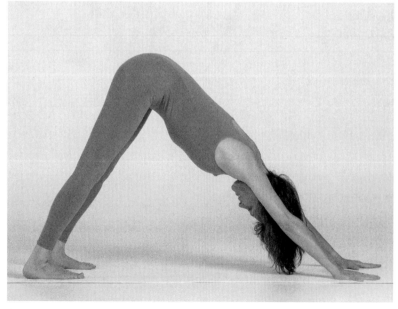

1

to the degree that allows you to maintain the length of your spine. Keep your leg muscles engaged to allow some areas to get stronger as you stretch your tight hamstrings and calves.

To come out, use the steps for the classic pose.

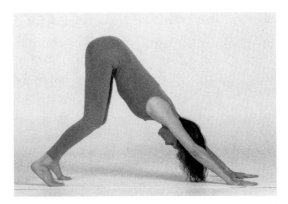

2

Version 3: Using a Chair

This is an alternative for those with wrist or hand problems and those who cannot get down to or up from the floor. This is also a good starting pose for people who are not yet strong enough for the classic pose.

Place a chair against a wall with the seat facing away from the wall. Stand a foot away from the chair and come into Standing Forward Bend, with your hands on the chair seat about shoulder distance apart. Depending on your comfort level, choose between hands flat on the seat or holding the edges. Then, bend your knees and walk your feet back away from the chair about three to four feet, lengthening from your hands to your hips in one straight line. Your legs can be straight or slightly bent, with heels on the floor or slightly lifted, while you float your head between your arms.

To come out, bend your knees and walk toward the chair. Then come up to Mountain Pose.

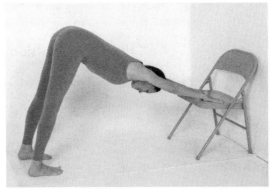

3

Version 4: Forearm Version

This is an alternative for those with wrist or hand problems that still provides full upper body strengthening for your upper arms, shoulders, chest, and back.

From a hands and knees position, place your elbows on the floor where your wrists were. Keep your hands and forearms in a parallel position, with palms down, about shoulder-width apart. Then lift your knees off the floor and push your hips up and back, away from your elbows, as you gradually straighten your legs. Press your forearms and hands forward into your mat and lengthen up and back from elbows to sitting bones. Because this version requires a lot of flexibility in your shoulders, start by holding it for short periods and work up to longer holds.

To come out, bring your knees back to the floor and come back into Child's Pose.

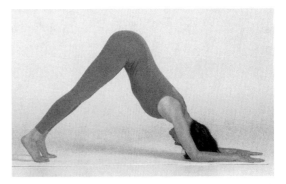

4

EASY SITTING POSE (*Sukhasana*)

This very accessible centering pose allows you to sit comfortably for meditation and breath practices and trains you to sit with good posture in other seated yoga poses and in everyday life. We prescribe this pose for posture, spine health, stiffness in the hips, stress, quieting the mind, and resting between other sitting poses.

CAUTIONS: If you have knee pain or hip pain in the pose and you've tried all four versions, try Hero Pose instead. If you can't get comfortable sitting on the ground for meditation or breath practice, sit on a chair instead. Those with lower back problems, herniated discs, or osteoporosis may need to avoid version 4.

Version 1: Classic Pose

Sit with your legs stretched out in front of you and your fingertips on the floor by your hips. Cross your legs, with your right shin in front of the left and your shins parallel with the front edge of your mat. Press your hands into the floor as you lengthen from your sitting bones to the crown of your head, creating an "inner lift." Tip your hips a bit forward to encourage the normal curve of your lower back and release your knees toward the floor. Maintaining your inner lift, rest your hands on your knees, relax your shoulder blades down, widen your collarbones, and align your head with your spine.

To come out, place your fingertips on the floor by your hips, lean back slightly, and extend your legs out in front of you. Alternate the cross of your legs from day to day.

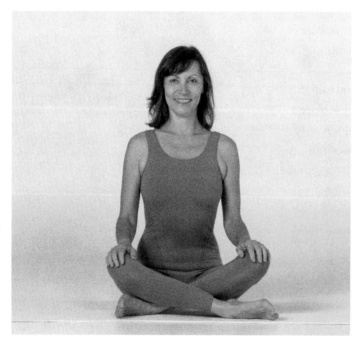

1

Version 2: Supported Hips and Knees

This is an alternative for those who cannot sit with good alignment in the classic pose.

Sit at the front edge of a prop, with sitting bones near its edge. (Experiment with the prop to find the height that allows you to experience the inner lift and spinal alignment described for the classic pose). Place blocks under your outer thighs so they fully support your thighs, using a height that allows you to relax your hip muscles and avoid knee or hip pain. Ankle support is optimal.

To come out, remove the props supporting your thighs and then use the steps for coming out of the classic pose.

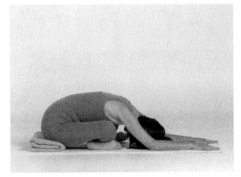

2

Version 3: Back against Wall

This is an alternative for those with weak back muscles or fatigue and an option for long seated meditations where you want extra support.

You can either use props as in version 2 or sit flat on the floor. If you are using a prop for your hips, place it against the wall. Now sit down on the floor or prop, with the back of your pelvis and shoulder blades against the wall, your lower back slightly off the wall, your head positioned over your shoulders, and your legs out in front of you. From here, follow the steps for the classic version.

To come out, use the steps for the classic pose or version 2 if you're using props.

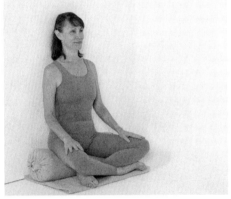

3

Version 4: Forward Bend

This is an option for stretching the muscles and fascia around your hips and along the sides of your spine. It's also effective for quieting the nervous system (although not for meditation or breath practice).

Start in version 1, 2, or 3. Maintaining a straight back and inner lift, tip forward from your hips and place your hands or fingertips on the floor in front of you. When your hips stop rotating forward, allow your lower spine to round a bit. Come forward gradually until you feel a good stretch in your hips, along your spine, or both. If you feel any pain in your knees, hips, or lower back, come slightly out of the pose until the pain disappears.

To come out, walk your hands back as you lift your spine back into an upright position. Change the cross of your legs and repeat on the other side.

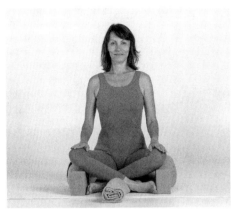

4

EASY SITTING TWIST (*Sukhasana* Twist)

This accessible, mildly stimulating pose improves your twisting ability while at the same time strengthening and stretching abdominal, chest, and back muscles and strengthening your spinal bones. We prescribe this pose for posture, spine health, fatigue, stimulating digestion, and as a counter pose for backbends and forward bends.

CAUTIONS: Those with osteoporosis should twist less deeply, as in version 4. For those with lower back pain, herniated discs, or sacroiliac problems, twists can worsen symptoms, so try version 4 or skip the pose. If your knees are painful in all versions, try practicing Reclined Twist instead.

Version 1: Classic Pose

Sit in Easy Sitting Pose, with your right shin in front of your left. With hands by your sides, press your fingers down to create an inner lift of your spine. Raise your arms up and out to your sides, parallel with the floor, then rotate your upper belly, chest, and head to the right. Place your left hand on your right knee and your right hand on the floor behind your hips. Concentrate your muscular action in your abdomen and spine instead of using your arms.

To come out, release the twist and return to center with your arms up and out to your sides. Then release your arms.

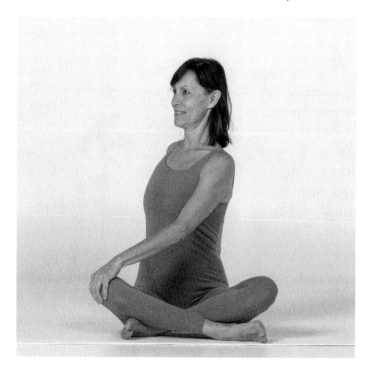

1

Version 2: Hand behind Back

This is an option for strengthening core muscles and stretching the shoulder of the back arm. (Those with shoulder injuries or rotator cuff problems may need to skip this.)

Follow the steps for the classic pose. Then, as you turn to your right, bend your right elbow, cross your right forearm around the back of your waist, and try to hook your right hand onto the top of your left thigh. If you can't take hold of your left thigh, press the back of your right hand as close to the left side of your waist as you can. Maintain a good inner lift of your spine.

To come out, use the steps for the classic pose.

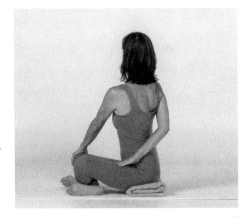

2

Version 3: Support for Hips

This is an alternative for those with tight hips and/or lower backs or who find it difficult to maintain a neutral spine while sitting flat on the floor.

Sit near the front edge of your prop (you can also prop your knees, as described in Easy Sitting Pose, version 2). Then follow the steps for the classic pose. If it is hard for you to reach the floor behind you or this causes you to lose the inner lift of your spine, add a low block behind your right hip to support your back hand.

To come out, use the steps for the classic pose.

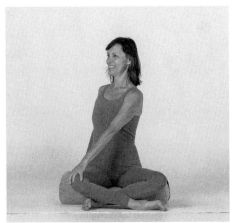

3

Version 4: Open Twist

This alternative is for those who should avoid the deeper twist of the classic pose, such as those with osteoporosis or mild lower back pain or who are in the second or third trimester of pregnancy.

Start in Easy Sitting Pose, with any propping as in version 3. Then come into the pose as in the classic version, but instead of bringing your left hand to your right knee as you twist to the right, simply rest it on your left knee. Turn more gently and not as deeply as you assess how your body handles the intensity of the twist.

To come out, use the steps for the classic pose.

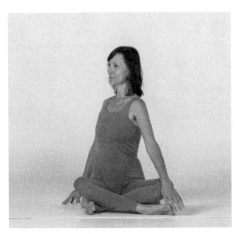

4

EXTENDED SIDE ANGLE POSE
(*Utthita Parsvakonasana*)

This energizing pose strengthens the muscles and bones in your legs, all along the sides of your torso, and around your shoulder joints while improving flexibility in your hips and shoulders. We prescribe this pose for fatigue, bone strength in hips and spine, balance, stress, and anxiety.

CAUTIONS: If you have lower back pain, a torn hamstring tendon, or sacroiliac problems and experience pain in the pose, come up higher or skip the pose. Those with knee problems should start with version 4 and use caution with the other versions. Those with shoulder problems/pain when the arm is overhead should place your hand on your hip instead. Because looking up toward the top arm can create neck pain, we recommend looking forward or down. Those with newly diagnosed or poorly controlled high blood pressure should hold the pose for only four breaths.

Version 1: Classic Pose

From Mountain Pose, step your feet about four to five feet apart. Turn your right foot and leg out 90 degrees, turn your back foot in about 10 degrees, and allow your hips to rotate slightly to the right without turning your chest. Lift your arms out to your sides then bend your right knee directly over your ankle to 90 degrees. Then side bend over your right thigh, bringing your right hand or fingers to the floor just to the outside of your right shin as you swing your left arm up and alongside your head. Encourage your belly and chest to rotate slightly upward but keep your head looking forward or at your front foot.

To come out, bring your torso up to vertical with your arms out to your sides as you straighten your bent knee. Then lower your arms and turn your feet to parallel.

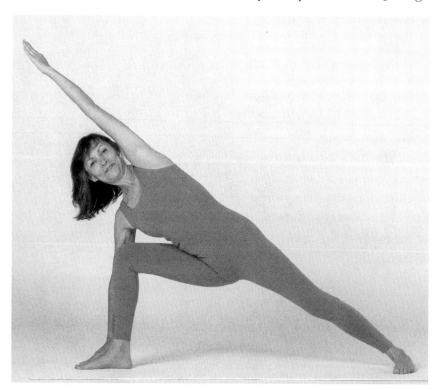

1

Version 2: Forearm on Thigh

This is an alternative for those who cannot do the classic pose with the hand on the floor or a block.

To come into the pose, use the steps for the classic pose until you have lifted your arms out to the sides (Warrior 2 Pose position). From Warrior 2 Pose, bend your right arm as you side bend over your right leg and place your forearm firmly on your thigh, near your knee. Press your forearm down as you lift up your right shoulder area, swing your left arm up and alongside your head, and rotate your chest.

To come out, use the steps for the classic pose.

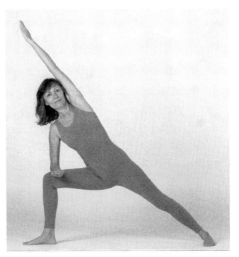

2

Version 3: Hand on Block

This alternative is for those who can't bring the hand to the floor in the classic pose but who find version 2 easy.

Try the block on its highest height first. If that's still too easy for you, experiment to find which height works best. Start with your feet wide apart as in the classic pose and place the block just to the outside of your right foot. When you come into the pose, bring your hand or fingertips to the block instead of down to the floor.

To come out, use the steps for the classic pose.

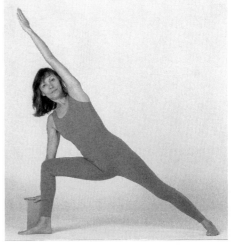

3

Version 4: Sitting on a Chair

This is an alternative for those who have weak legs or knee or hip pain when bearing full weight on a bent knee or for those with balance problems.

Place the chair on the center of your mat, with the front of the chair seat facing the long edge of your mat and with only the front legs on the mat. Sit on the front edge of the chair seat, with your knees bent and your feet flat on the floor. Swing your right leg 90 degrees to the right, keeping the knee bent and letting the chair seat support your right sitting bone and the back of your thigh. Extend your left leg out straight to your left, a bit forward of your right leg. Bring your arms up and out to your sides, parallel with floor. Then, as you tip down, bend your elbow, and place your forearm firmly on your thigh, near your knee, as you bring your left arm up and alongside your head.

To come out, lift your torso back up to vertical and your arms out to your sides. Then bend your left knee, bring both legs together in front of you, and release your arms to your sides.

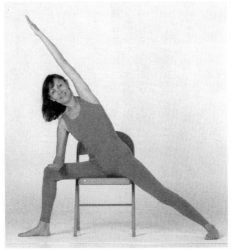

4

HALF DOWNWARD-FACING DOG POSE
(*Ardha Adho Mukha Svanasana*)

This fantastic allover stretch opens your shoulders and stretches your arms, back, chest, spine, and legs, making it a wonderful warm-up pose and an excellent way to start a practice. We prescribe this pose for lower back pain, spine health, stress, improving breath capacity, and as an alternative to Downward-Facing Dog Pose.

CAUTIONS: Those with lower back pain should try version 2 or 4. If you have wrist pain, place your fingertips or fists on the wall instead of your palms. If you have a shoulder injury or shoulder pain, straighten your arms cautiously, going only as far as you can without pain. Those with abdominal hernias or women with abdominal wall separation should start with short holds.

Version 1: Classic Pose

Stand facing a wall, about one foot away. With your arms at your sides, bend your elbows to 90 degrees and place your palms flat on the wall directly in front of your elbows, with forearms parallel to floor. Bend your knees and push your sitting bones away from the wall. Then press your hands firmly into the wall and slowly walk your feet away from it, keeping your hips directly above your heels. Stop when your arms and torso make one long line, parallel to the floor, with your legs straight, feet hip-distance apart, and head even between your ears.

To come out, bend your knees and slowly walk forward to standing. Then shake out your wrists.

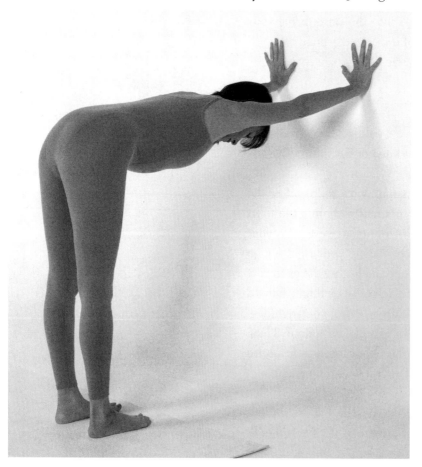

1

Version 2: Bent Knees

This is an alternative for those who are flexible in the shoulders but have stiff legs or who experience lower back pain in the classic pose.

To come into the pose, use the steps for the classic pose, but when your pelvis is over your feet, keep your knees slightly bent, so you feel a bit of stretching in the backs of your legs, but no pain in your lower back. (If you feel pain, try bending your knees even more or practice version 4.)

To come out, use the steps for the classic pose.

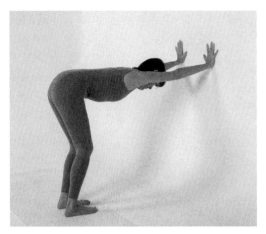

2

Version 3: Higher Hands

This alternative is for those who can easily do version 2 but cannot do the classic pose without shoulder discomfort or pain or those who feel intense stretching in their legs in the classic pose.

To come into the pose, stand facing a wall, about one foot away. Place your hands on the wall in front of your shoulders, about shoulder-width apart (higher than in the classic pose). Then press your hands into the wall and walk your feet away from the wall, stopping when your pelvis is directly over your feet, and your arms and torso are slightly angled, forming a long, even line. Straighten your legs and use the steps for the classic pose for aligning your feet and head.

To come out, use the steps for the classic pose.

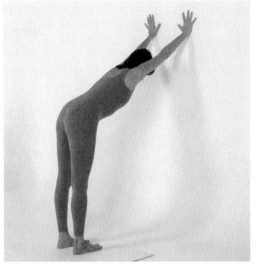

3

Version 4: Higher Hands with Bent Knees

This is an alternative for those who have tight shoulders, very tight legs, or lower back pain and cannot comfortably practice other versions.

To come into the pose, place your hands on the wall in front of your shoulders and about shoulder-width apart, as in version 3. Bend your knees and push your sitting bones away from the wall. Then press your hands firmly into the wall and slowly walk your feet away from the wall, stopping as soon as you feel your shoulders tighten or notice any pain. Keep your knees slightly bent and your leg muscles strong. Use the steps for the classic pose for aligning your feet and head.

To come out, use the steps for the classic pose.

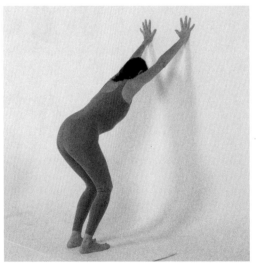

4

HERO POSE (*Virasana*)

This stable, centering seated pose is suitable for meditation and breath practices, strengthens the back muscles needed to support your spine in a healthy position, and stretches the fronts of your thighs, shins, and ankles. We prescribe this pose for posture, spine health, stress, quieting the mind, and preparing for backbends.

CAUTIONS: Come out of the pose if your feet or legs feel numb or tingly. If you have knee pain in the pose and have tried all four versions, try sitting on an even higher prop or practice Easy Sitting Pose instead.

Version 1: Classic Pose

This version is for those who can sit without a prop with no pain while maintaining the natural curve of the lower spine.

Kneel on a folded blanket, with knees near the front of the blanket and ankles and feet hanging off the back edge, toes pointing straight back. Position your legs so your knees are hip-distance apart but your shins are a bit wider apart in back. Slowly bring your sitting bones down between your feet. If needed, adjust your pelvis until your lower back is in its natural curve. Place your fingertips on the floor outside your hips and press them down as you lengthen from your sitting bones to the crown of your head, creating an "inner lift." Rest your hands on your knees, relax your shoulder blades down, widen your collarbones, and align your head with your spine.

To come out, lift your hips up and reach your hands forward to come into hands and knees position. From there, stretch one leg out behind you, then repeat with the other leg.

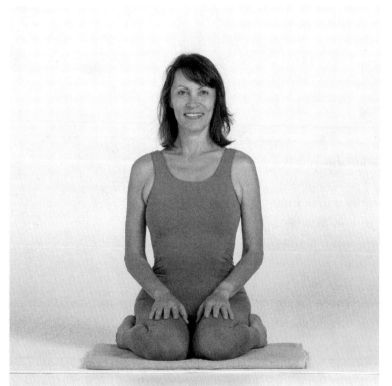

1

Version 2: On a Block

This is an alternative for those with tight knees or front thigh muscles, or for those with a rounded lower back in the classic pose, and an option for anyone who wants to sit for longer sessions.

Kneel on a folded blanket as in the classic pose and place a block on its lowest or middle height (or use a stack of two blocks) sideways between your feet, so you'll be able to rest both sitting bones on it. Then slowly bring your sitting bones onto the block. If there is any pain in your hips, thighs, knees, or ankles, come up again and try a higher prop. Use the steps for the classic pose to find your inner lift.

To come out, lift your hips and remove the prop. Then come onto hands and knees to stretch your legs.

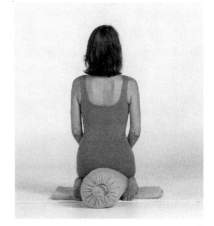

2

Version 3: On a Bolster

This is an option for those who need or want a more comfortable and slightly higher prop than the one used in version 2, particularly for longer sitting sessions.

Place a bolster lengthwise on your mat with your folded blanket in front of it. Kneel in front of the end of the bolster, so it lies between your ankles. Then slowly bring your sitting bones onto the bolster. If there is any pain in your hips, thighs, knees, or ankles, try placing a block on its lowest height under the front of the bolster. Use the steps for the classic pose to find your inner lift.

To come out, lift your hips and remove the bolster between your feet. Then come onto hands and knees to stretch your legs.

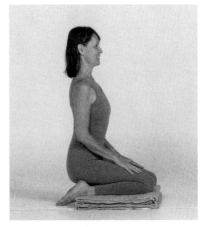

3

Version 4: Support for Ankles

This alternative is for those with stiff or painful ankles or who can't get comfortable in version 2 or 3.

Stack two, three, or more blankets on your mat. If you normally sit on a prop, place the prop near the back edge of the blanket stack. Kneel on the blanket stack with your ankles at the very back edge of the blankets and your feet hanging off. Then lower your sitting bones onto either the blanket stack or the prop. If you have any pain in your ankles, try adding yet another blanket to your stack. Use the steps for the classic pose to find your inner lift.

To come out, lift your hips, place your hands on the floor, and move the props. Then come onto your hands and knees to stretch your legs.

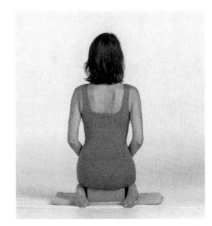

4

HUNTING DOG POSE

This mildly stimulating pose strengthens your upper body, as well as your pelvic and core belly muscles, and helps improve balance and coordination. We prescribe this pose for lower back pain, fatigue, bone strength for wrists and spine, and concentration.

CAUTIONS: If you have lower back pain, start with version 2 or 3 and progress from there. If you have wrist pain, try coming onto your fingertips, making fists, or coming down onto your forearms with your shoulders over your elbows. If you have a shoulder injury or shoulder pain, take your arm out only as far as you can without pain. Those with newly diagnosed or poorly controlled high blood pressure should hold the full pose for only four breaths.

Version 1: Classic Pose

Place a folded blanket across the middle of your mat and come onto your hands and knees, with your knees on the blanket, and your hands and the tops of your feet on the mat. Maintaining a neutral spine from your tailbone to the crown of your head, strengthen your arms. Then mindfully straighten your right leg behind you, with your toes turned under and the ball of your foot on floor. Keeping your pelvis and lower back stable, raise your right leg until it is about parallel with the floor. Firm your right arm, and as you press down into your right hand, lift your breastbone away from the floor. Then lift your left arm forward and up to be parallel with the floor.

To come out, return your left hand and right knee to the floor. Lift your right hand up, and shake out your right hand and wrist.

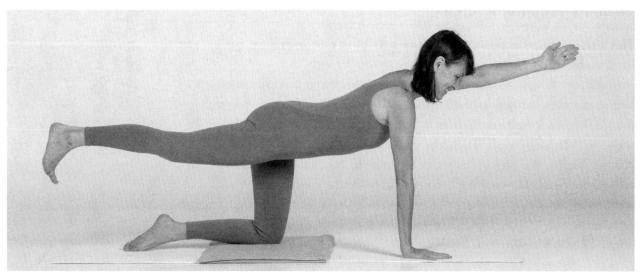

1

Version 2: Foot on Floor

This is an alternative for those with active lower back pain or general weakness and an option to prepare for versions 1 and 4.

Use the steps for the classic pose for setting up, coming onto your hands and knees, and lengthening your right leg behind you. With your foot lightly touching the floor, keep pressing down both hands into the floor as you lift your breastbone away from it. Imagine you are slightly lifting up your back leg.

To come out, return your right knee to the floor. Shake out your hands and wrists.

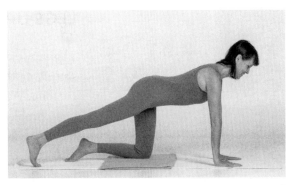

2

Version 3: Arm Only

This is an alternative for those with general weakness, those who want to work only on upper body strength and balance, and those who experience back pain in version 1, 2, or 4.

Use the steps for the classic pose for setting up and coming onto your hands and knees. Maintaining a neutral spine from your tailbone to the crown of your head, strengthen your left arm, pressing down into your left hand as you lift your breastbone away from the floor. Then raise your right arm forward and up so it is parallel to the floor.

To come out, bring your left hand back to the floor. Shake out your right hand and wrist.

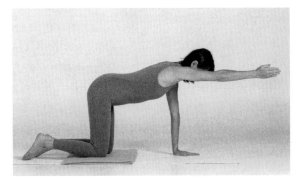

3

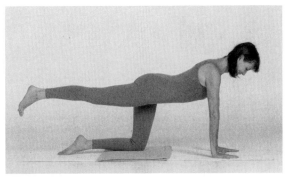

4

Version 4: Leg Only

This is an alternative for those who do not have enough strength to do the classic pose and for those who have shoulder pain in versions 1 and 3.

Use the steps for the classic pose for setting up, coming onto your hands and knees, and lifting your right leg. Maintaining a neutral spine from your tailbone to the crown of your head, strengthen your arms and press down into both hands as you lift your breastbone away from the floor. Lengthen from the crown of your head to your right heel.

To come out, return your right knee to the floor, and one at a time shake out your hands and wrists.

LEGS UP THE WALL POSE (*Viparita Karani*)

This very calming inverted pose triggers the relaxation response while also stretching the backs of your legs, opening your chest, and improving circulation. We prescribe this pose for lower back pain, circulation, foot and knee problems, stress, fatigue, anxiety, insomnia, calming digestion, and quieting the mind.

CAUTIONS: Come into the pose slowly to avoid quickly dropping your head. Do not roll your head from side to side in this pose, as this could injure your neck. Those with symptomatic hiatal hernia, acid reflux, sinus congestion, or allergy drainage may not be able to lie flat, so try keeping your hips on the floor and adding a prop under your torso, or skip the pose entirely. Those with back pain may need to bend the knees slightly, move farther away from the wall, or do version 4 of Relaxation Pose instead.

Version 1: Classic Pose

Place a bolster on the mat about six inches away from the wall and parallel to it. Sit on the end of the bolster, sideways to the wall, with your knees bent and your feet on the floor. Then swivel toward the wall, extending your legs up the wall as you use your hands to slowly lower your back and head to the floor. Center your pelvis on the top of the bolster and straighten your legs, with your heels resting on the wall. Bring your arms into a cactus position by your ears or relax them by your sides. Close your eyes and practice simple breath awareness or any other meditation technique.

To come out, slide your feet down the wall and bend your knees toward your chest. Then, gently roll to one side to come off the bolster and use your hands to slowly press yourself up to a sitting position, resting for a few breaths.

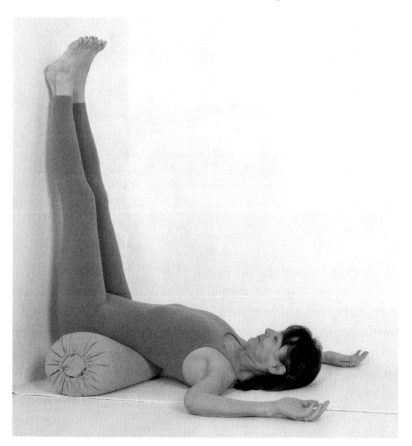

1

Version 2: Pelvis on Blanket

This alternative is for those who feel lower back pain in the classic pose or for those who just prefer this version. This is also an option for a more intense leg stretch.

Fold a blanket into a long, narrow rectangle that is about the same length and width as a bolster. Then place the folded blanket on a mat about six inches from the wall. To come into the pose, sit on the end of the blanket sideways to the wall, with your knees bent and the soles of your feet on the floor. Then use the steps for entering the classic pose, adjusting the position of your pelvis and blanket if needed.

To come out, use the steps for the classic pose.

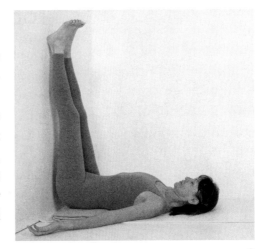

2

Version 3: No Pelvic Support

This is an alternative for those who don't feel comfortable using a prop or who don't have one. It's also a good option for resting your lower back.

To come into the pose, sit sideways to the wall, about six inches away, with your knees bent and the soles of your feet on the floor. Then use the steps for entering the classic pose. After you're up, you can shift your pelvis closer to or farther from the wall if necessary.

To come out, use the steps for the classic pose.

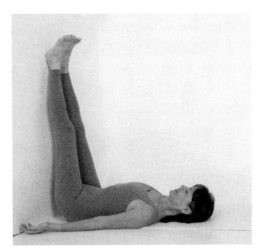

3

Version 4: Easy Inverted Pose

This is an alternative for those who have lower back or leg pain or who just can't get comfortable in the classic pose.

Place a chair at one end of your mat, facing the other end, with a folded blanket on the seat. Fold one or two blankets into long, thin rectangles and place them cross-wise on the mat, about a foot away from the chair. Sitting on the end of the rectangular blankets, sideways to the chair, swing your calves up onto the chair seat, extending your feet through the chair back if needed, and use your hands to guide your back and head to the floor. If your calves are not resting comfortably, adjust the position of your hips (and the prop).

To come out, bring your knees toward your chest, placing your feet on the front edge of the chair. Then follow the steps for the classic pose.

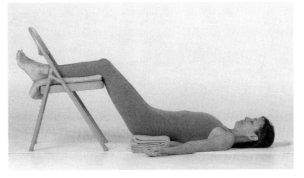

4

LOCUST POSE (*Salabhasana*)

This basic, accessible backbend strengthens your entire back body, from the nape of your neck to the backs of your heels, as well as your arms. We prescribe this pose for lower back pain, posture, fatigue, bone strength in spine, spine health, and depression.

CAUTIONS: If you feel cramps in your feet, hamstrings, or lower back, try lowering down a bit or come up more slowly. Those with back pain should start with version 3 and gradually progress to the classic pose. Those with abdominal hernias or women with abdominal wall separation should practice this pose with care so it does not worsen your condition, or try Bridge Pose instead. Those with newly diagnosed or poorly controlled high blood pressure should hold the pose for only four breaths.

Version 1: Classic Pose

Lie on your belly, with your arms by your sides, palms down, and your forehead or chin on the floor. Turn your palms to face up and create a sense of length from your hips into your feet and from your tailbone up to the crown of your head. With your pelvis and lower belly on the floor, inhale and lift your chest, head, and legs just a few inches off the floor, and raise your arms to be parallel with the floor. Keeping your knees straight, lengthen your legs back as you reach forward through the crown of your head.

To come out, release your legs, chest, head, and arms, returning to the starting position.

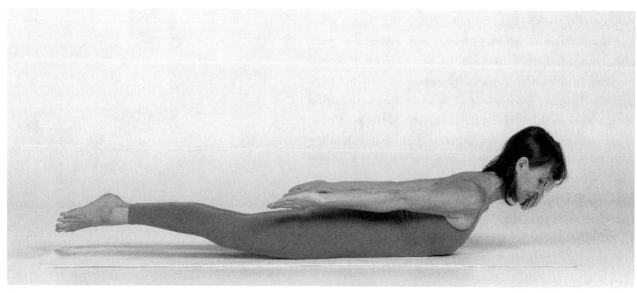

1

Version 2: Bolster under Chest, Legs on the Floor

This is an easier alternative for people who are stiff or weak in the upper chest and an option for focusing on the chest opening.

Lie with the bolster crosswise under your lower ribs, with your arms behind you alongside your hips and your palms facing up, and with your head and neck relaxed. Inhale as you roll your head and chest up into a backbend, lifting your arms up to be parallel with the floor and widening your collarbones. Keep your legs on the floor but activate and lengthen them.

To come out, release your chest, head, and arms and drape them over the bolster. Then use your hands to push yourself back off the bolster.

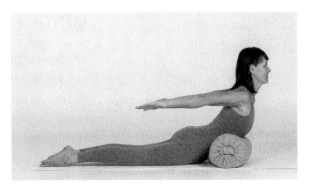

2

Version 3: One Leg at a Time, Palms Down

This alternative is for those with back problems as it strengthens the lower back muscles in an easier version of the pose.

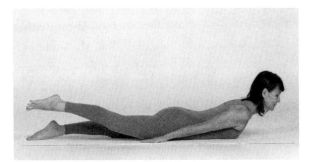

3

After creating a sense of length in your starting position, keep your hips evenly aligned on the floor as you inhale and come into the pose. Roll your head and chest up a few inches and lift your arms up to be parallel with the floor (palms facing up) or keep them on the floor (palms facing down). Lift your right leg up a few inches while continuing to lengthen both legs toward your toes. Keep your front hips even on the floor.

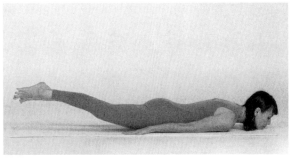

4

To come out, release your leg, chest, head, and arms, returning to the starting position. Rest for a few breaths before repeating on the left.

Version 4: Legs Only, Palms Down

This option allows you to focus on strengthening your lower back, legs, and buttocks.

Take the starting position for the classic pose with palms facing down. Create a sense of length as you lift up your legs a few inches while keeping your torso, arms, and chin or forehead on the floor. Pressing your hands into the floor, try to swing your legs an inch or two higher. Since this takes extra effort, start with shorter holds and work up gradually to longer holds.

To come out, release your legs, returning to the starting position.

LUNGE POSE (*Vanarasana*)

This energizing pose lengthens and strengthens the muscles around your hip joints, stretches your calf muscles, and strengthens your arms and upper chest. We prescribe this pose for lower back pain, bone strength in hips, arthritis of hips, balance, and preparing for standing poses and backbends.

CAUTIONS: Those with sacroiliac problems should keep your pelvis in a neutral alignment. Anyone with hamstring or groin pulls should wait until completely healed before doing this pose. Those with knee pain should use blocks or a chair to lessen the compression of your front knee. Those with newly diagnosed or poorly controlled high blood pressure should hold the pose for only four breaths.

Version 1: Classic Pose

From Mountain Pose, come into an easy Standing Forward Bend, with fingertips on the floor. Bend your knees and step your left foot back far enough so you can straighten your left leg while keeping your right knee over your right ankle. Keep the ball of your left foot on the ground, toes pointing forward. Position your arms parallel with your front shinbone and press your fingers or hands down as you lengthen your arms up toward your shoulders. Lengthen from your left heel through your left leg and spine and out to the top of your head and lengthen the front of your body from your pubic bone to your collarbones.

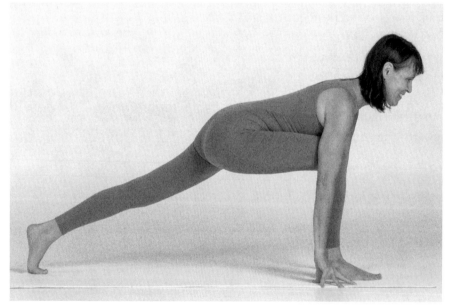

1

To come out, bend your back knee slightly and step forward into Standing Forward Bend. From there, lift up to Mountain Pose.

Version 2: Hands on Blocks

This alternative is for those with stiff hips, knee pain with a deep bend of the front knee, shorter arms, or a larger chest.

Stand in Mountain Pose and place the blocks at the height you prefer near the outer edges of your feet. Then follow the steps for the classic pose, bringing your hands onto the blocks in both Standing Forward Bend and Lunge Pose, so when you're in the lunge, the blocks are just outside your shins and directly under your shoulders. (Move the blocks if necessary.)

To come out, bend your back knee slightly and step forward into Standing Forward Bend. From there, lift up to Mountain Pose.

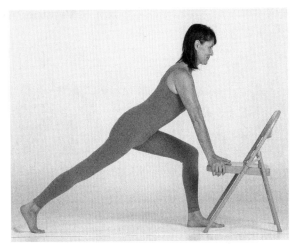

2

Version 3: Hands on Chair

This is a gentle alternative for those with stiff hips, knees, or spines. It's also good for those with balance problems.

Place a chair at the front of your mat so it faces you. Stand a foot away from the chair. Release into Standing Forward Bend, with your hands or fingers on the front of the chair seat. Step your right foot back into classic Lunge Pose, aligning your front knee over your ankle joint. Keep your arms straight and strong, your spine long, and your back knee engaged.

To come out, bend your back knee slightly then step your back foot forward to match your front foot. From there, lift up to Mountain Pose.

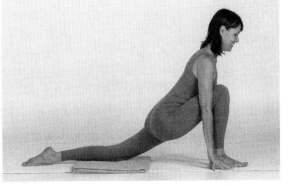

3

Version 4: Dropped Knee

This option stretches the front hip muscles of your back leg (a good warm-up for backbends) and provides a deeper stretch for the back of your front hip and upper leg.

Place a folded blanket across the center of your mat. Move into the classic pose, stepping your back foot over the blanket. From there, bend your back knee and gently lower it down to the blanket. With the tops of your back toes on the floor, shift your hips slightly forward in space until you feel a stretch in your back hip joint. Keep your arms active and spine long. Use blocks for your hands if needed.

To come out, turn your back toes under, straighten your back leg, and step your back foot forward into Standing Forward Bend. From there, lift up to Mountain Pose.

4

MOUNTAIN POSE (*Tadasana*)

This grounding pose is the ideal, active standing posture, teaching you healthy alignment of pelvis and spine over feet and head over torso, while cultivating strong legs and an even opening in your chest and upper back. We prescribe this pose for lower back pain, posture, balance, spine health, and as a resting pose between standing poses.

CAUTIONS: This pose is generally very safe and accessible. If you have trouble with balance, step your feet wider apart and/or practice with your back near a wall.

Version 1: Classic Pose

Stand with your feet parallel and hip-distance apart. Distribute your weight evenly on your feet and firm your upper thigh muscles toward your thighbones. From your tailbone, lengthen upward through your spine to the crown of your head, as if growing taller. Without squeezing your shoulder blades together, widen both the front of your chest and your upper back. Position your head directly over your shoulders, with your chin parallel with the floor. Either relax your arms at your sides or actively reach down from your shoulders into your fingers, with palms facing your thighs.

To come out, simply relax your physical effort and notice the posture your body returns to.

Version 2: Block between Thighs

This is an option for strengthening and bringing awareness to your legs, especially your inner thigh muscles.

Start in the classic pose. Place a block at its narrowest width between your thighs, halfway between your pelvis and inner knees. Step your feet a bit closer together, firming your legs into the block while lengthening down into your feet. If you tend to flatten your lower back, roll your thighs in and push the block back slightly to encourage a normal lumbar curve. If you have a swayback that is painful, squeeze the block and draw your tailbone down slightly toward the block. Follow the leg, spine, chest, and head instructions for the classic pose.

To come out, remove the block and relax your physical effort, especially your legs.

Version 3: Reverse Prayer Position

This option opens the front of your chest and shoulder joints, strengthens the muscles between your shoulder blades, and stretches your forearms and wrists.

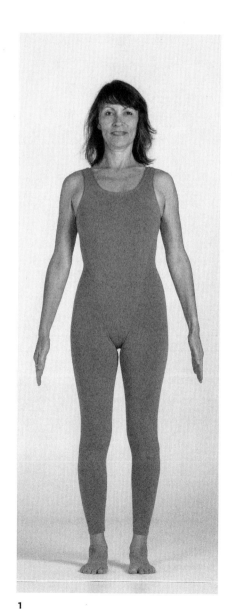

1

Start in the classic pose. Bring your palms together into Prayer position in front of your chest and press your palms together. Release your hands and, keeping your elbows bent, bring your palms together behind your back, with fingertips pointing down. Move your hands a few inches away from your lower back and spin your fingertips up toward your head. With the pinky sides of your hands lightly touching your lower back, wriggle your hands up your spine as high as you can comfortably go, with palms and thumbs together if possible.

To come out, carefully wiggle your hands down at least six inches and release them by your sides. Shake out your hands and arms.

Version 4: Elbows Clasped Behind Back

This is an alternative to version 3 for those who cannot bring their palms together.

Follow the steps for version 3 but instead of bringing your palms together behind your back, bring just your right arm behind your back. Then bring your left arm back and, depending on your flexibility, clasp either opposite elbows or forearms.

To come out, release your arms. Repeat the arm position on the left side by taking your left arm back first. After finishing both sides, shake out your arms.

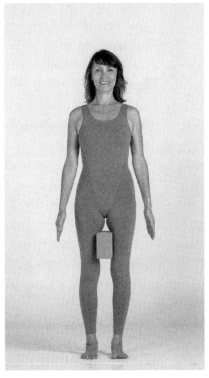

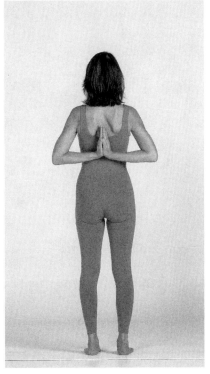

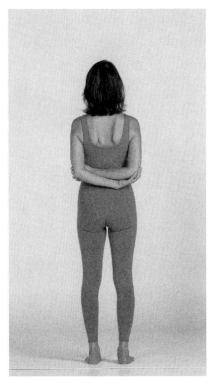

2

3

4

PLANK POSE (*Phalankasana*)

This active, challenging pose is very strengthening, building shoulder girdle strength and stability, abdominal/core and arm strength, and leg strength. We prescribe this pose for bone strength in the wrists and spine, concentration, and cultivating equanimity.

CAUTIONS: Those with wrist problems or hand pain should try version 2. Those with abdominal hernias or women with separation of the abdominal wall should start with short holds. Those with newly diagnosed or poorly controlled high blood pressure should hold the pose for only four breaths.

Version 1: Classic Pose

Start in the classic Downward-Facing Dog Pose. Shift your body forward, bringing your shoulders directly over your wrist joints. Keep your head in line with your spine. Draw a mental line from your shoulders to your heels and check if your hips are higher or lower than that line. If so, adjust the position of your feet. Firm your elbow joints, lifting from your wrists to your shoulders, and lift your breastbone away from the floor to stabilize your shoulders. Firm your leg muscles and firm your belly up toward your spine without flattening your lower back.

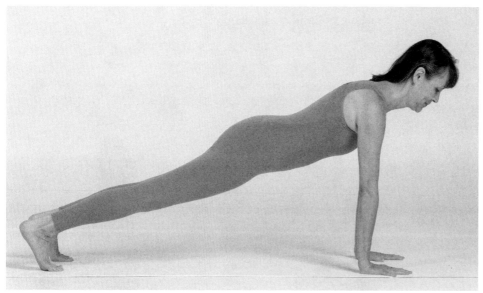

1

To come out, shift back to Downward-Facing Dog Pose and release your knees to the floor. Then shake out your hands and wrists.

Version 2: On Forearms

This alternative is for those who have wrist or hand problems. It's also an option for targeting upper body and abdominal strength.

Start in version 4 of Downward-Facing Dog Pose. Shift your shoulders forward so they are directly over your elbows. If necessary, wiggle your feet back two to six inches until your hips come in line with your shoulders and heels. Keep your head in line with your spine. Press the entire length of your forearms into the floor, so your weight does not drop heavily on your elbow joints.

To come out, shift back to version 4 of Downward-Facing Dog Pose and release your knees to the floor. Then shake out your hands and wrists.

Version 3: On a Chair

This is an easy alternative for beginners and those with less strength. It's also a possible alternative for those with wrist problems.

Place the back of a chair against a wall and come into version 3 of Downward-Facing Dog Pose. With straight arms, shift your body forward until your shoulders are over your wrists and your body forms a straight line from your lifted heels through your hips to your shoulders. Keep your head in line with your spine.

To come out, shift your hips back to Downward-Facing Dog Pose, then bend your knees and walk forward to come into Mountain Pose. Then shake out your hands and wrists.

Version 4: Knees Down

This is an alternative for beginners or those who are moving toward the classic pose. It's also a substitute for Upward-Facing Dog Pose or Cobra Pose in Sun Salutations.

Place a folded blanket in the middle of your mat. Then come briefly into the classic pose. Bend your knees and release them to the floor. With knees touching down, lift your shinbones up toward the ceiling and bring your hips in line with your knees and shoulders, maintaining a shoulders-over-the-wrists alignment. Move your hands forward or back a few inches if necessary.

To come out, push yourself back into Child's Pose. Then shake out your hands and wrists.

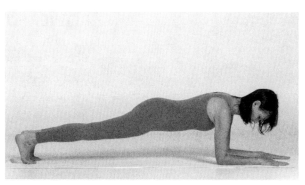

2

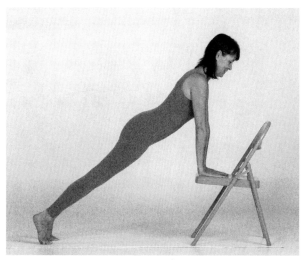

3

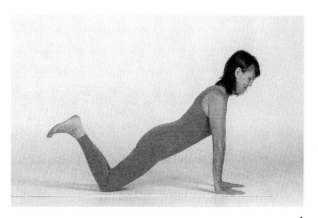

4

POWERFUL POSE (*Utkatasana*)

This accessible, energizing pose strengthens your leg, arm, and upper back muscles, while stretching your chest, shoulders, and arms. We prescribe this pose for posture, fatigue, balance, and preparing for bent-knee standing poses.

CAUTIONS: Those with knee pain should avoid deeply bending your knees, going only as far as is comfortable. Those with lower back pain should keep your spine more upright. If you have a shoulder injury or shoulder pain, take your arms up only as far as you can without pain or try version 4. Those with newly diagnosed or poorly controlled high blood pressure should hold the pose for only four breaths.

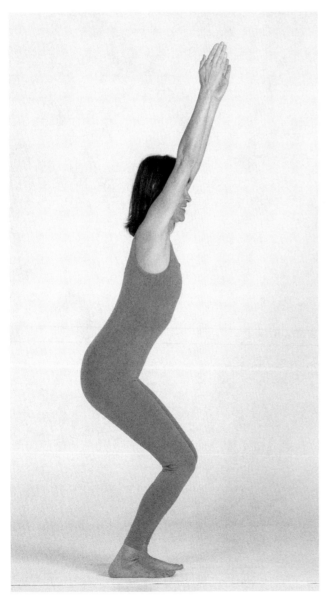

Version 1: Classic Pose

Start in Mountain Pose with your feet parallel and hip-distance apart. Swing your arms forward and up, alongside your ears. Aim your knees straight forward and bend them a few inches while keeping your heels on the floor. Maintaining a Mountain Pose spine, bend from your hips to tip your torso forward a few inches. Firm your leg muscles and energize your arms, reaching from the sides of your waist through your fingertips while keeping your head in a neutral position between your arms.

To come out, straighten your legs. Then release your arms to your sides.

Version 2: Block between Thighs

This option provides more strengthening of your inner leg and deep abdominal muscles.

Standing in Mountain Pose, place a block on its narrowest or middle width about halfway between your knees and your pelvis. Then squeeze the block firmly with your inner thigh muscles and adjust your feet so they are parallel and in line with the center of your hip joints. Bend your knees and raise your arms as in the classic pose while continuing to squeeze the block.

To come out, continue to squeeze the block as you straighten your legs. Then release your arms.

Version 3: Hips on Wall

This is an easier alternative for those with poor balance or weak legs.

Start in Mountain Pose with your back to a wall about one foot away. Follow the steps for the classic pose, but as you tip your torso forward, move your buttocks back to rest against the wall. Maintaining contact with the wall, work your legs and arms as in the classic pose.

To come out, release your arms to your sides and place your hands on the wall beside your hips. Straighten your legs and use your hands to push yourself gently forward into Mountain Pose.

Version 4: Hands on Hips

This alternative is for those with shoulder problems and those who have trouble balancing in the classic pose.

Start in Mountain Pose with your hands on your hips. Then enter the pose by bending your knees and tipping your torso forward as in the classic pose. Keeping your spine in a neutral position, firm your leg muscles and release your shoulder blades down your back. Keep your head in a neutral position, aligned with your spine.

To come out, straighten your legs and release your arms to your sides, returning to Mountain Pose.

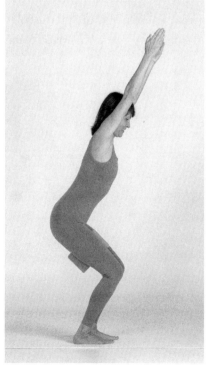

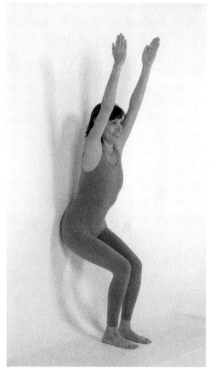

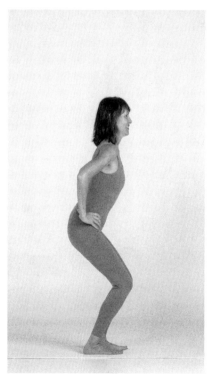

2   3   4

RECLINED COBBLER'S POSE
(*Supta Baddha Konasana*)

This quieting restorative pose relaxes you when you're stressed and re-freshes you when you're fatigued, while also providing a gentle stretch for your front body, spine, and hips. We prescribe this pose for stress, fatigue, depression, insomnia, quieting the digestive system, and quieting the mind.

CAUTIONS: Make sure you don't fall asleep in the pose for long periods of time, as you can overstretch. Those with back pain may need to sit farther away from the support under your torso. Those with shoulder problems can try placing folded blankets under your arms. Those with hip or knee pain in the pose should use higher props under your legs.

Version 1: Classic Pose

Fold one or two blankets lengthwise into long rectangles about four to six inches wide, about the size of a bolster. Then lay the blanket or blanket stack lengthwise on your mat. Sit in front of the narrow edge (not on it) and come into Cobbler's Pose, version 1. Slowly lower your torso and head onto the prop without lifting your buttocks off the mat. To support your head, fold the far end of the top blanket under or add another blanket, as shown. Bring your arms out to your sides, at a 45- to 90-degree angle, with palms facing up.

To come out, use your hands to bring your knees together and the soles of your feet to the floor. Then roll to one side and use your hands to come up to sitting. Sit quietly for a few breaths.

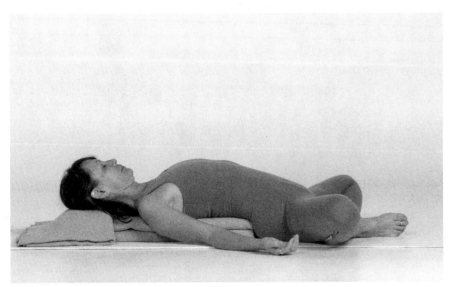

1

Version 2: Elevated Bolster

This is an alternative for those with tight hips or difficulty with back bending. This is also an option for a more relaxing experience.

Place a bolster lengthwise along your mat, adding one or two blocks underneath it to create a sloping angle. We also recommend adding a folded blanket at the end to support your head. Then sit in front of the bolster (not on it), come into Cobbler's Pose, version 1, and use your hands to lower yourself onto the bolster. If your hips or knees are uncomfortable, support them with blocks or rolled blankets. Position your arms as in the classic pose.

To come out, use the steps for the classic pose.

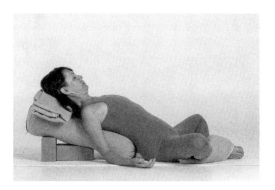

2

Version 3: Support for Hips and Knees

This is an alternative for those with tight hips, painful knees, sacroiliac joint problems, or discomfort in your legs.

Use the setup for the classic pose or version 2. When you come into Cobbler's Pose, version 1, slip blocks or rolled blankets under your knees and upper thighs and release your legs completely onto the supports. If you can't relax your legs completely or you're still not comfortable, try higher supports or reposition the props to find the optimum support.

To come out, use the steps for the classic pose.

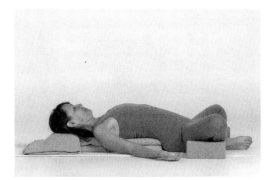

3

Version 4: Calves on a Chair

This is an alternative for those with back or hip pain or discomfort and those who cannot do Legs Up the Wall Pose.

Place your chair on the front of your mat, with the seat facing the back. Place a mat or folded blanket on the seat. Lie on your back in front of the chair with your calves resting comfortably on the seat. Then release your knees apart into Cobbler's Pose, allowing your feet to separate until the outer sides of your lower legs are resting comfortably. If your lower legs are not relaxing, scoot yourself farther forward or back.

To come out, bring your knees together and your feet to the edge of the seat. Then roll to one side as you gently lower your feet and legs to the floor and use your hands to come up to sitting.

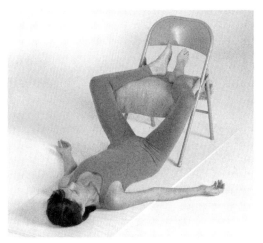

4

RECLINED LEG STRETCH
(*Supta Padangusthasana*)

This versatile stretching pose has four versions that stretch your hips in several directions while also stretching the backs of your legs and lengthening your lower back. We prescribe this pose for lower back pain, stress, arthritis of hips and knees, knee problems, and preparing the hips for standing poses, seated poses, and twists.

CAUTIONS: If you experience lower back pain in versions 1 or 2, bend your bottom leg and place the foot on the floor. If lower back pain is an ongoing problem, skip version 4 entirely. For any version, if the pose causes hip or back pain, try backing off a bit to see if the pain resolves. If not, skip that version.

Version 1: Leg Straight Up

This version stretches the back of your hip and all the muscles in the back of your top leg, providing relief from lower back pain.

From version 4 of Relaxation Pose, bring your right knee into your chest, place a strap over the arch of your right foot, and stretch your right foot toward the ceiling. Walk both hands up the sides of the strap until your arms are straight, and lengthen your left leg along the ground. Adjust your right leg forward or back until you can easily straighten your right knee and still feel a stretch. Relax your shoulders and make sure your lower spine is either softly touching the floor or slightly arched away from it.

To come out, bend your right knee, slip the strap off your foot, lower your right leg to the floor, and bend both knees. Shake out your hands and wrists.

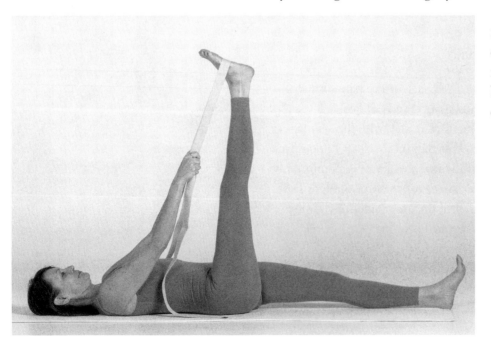

1

Version 2: Leg to the Side

This version focuses the stretch on the inner thigh muscles of your raised leg and strengthens your core muscles, which helps relieve lower back pain by improving spinal stability.

Start in version 1. Then take both sides of the strap into your right hand and stretch your left arm out to your left side in a *T* position. Stretch through your left leg as you slowly bring your right leg out to your right side and down toward the floor, stopping when your foot is one to two feet from the floor. Bring your right elbow to the floor as you keep tension on the strap and press your right foot into it. If holding your leg out to the side is painful or difficult, place a prop under your right thigh.

To come out, return to version 1 by lifting your leg back to vertical. Then use the steps for coming out of version 1.

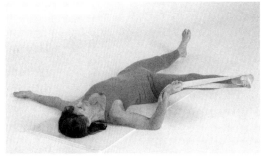

2

Version 3: Scissor Legs

This version concentrates the stretch on your outer hip and leg. Because it doesn't require twisting, it is safer than version 4 for someone with lower back pain.

Start in version 1. Then take both sides of the strap into your left hand and extend your right arm out to the side in a *T* position. Keeping your lower back and pelvis on the floor, bring your right leg toward your left, about six to twelve inches across the midline of your body. Keep some tension on the strap and press your right foot into it.

To come out, return to version 1 by bringing your leg back to vertical. Then use the steps for coming out of version 1.

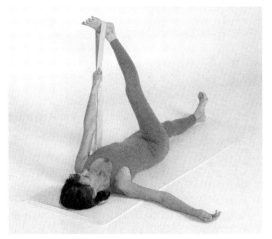

3

Version 4: Twisting

This version focuses the stretch on your outer hip and leg along with your deep buttock muscles, while also opening your chest and releasing tight back muscles.

Start in version 1. Then take both sides of the strap into your left hand and extend your right arm out to the side in a *T* position. Roll your hips and legs to the left, coming onto your outer left leg so your right hip is stacked on the left. Swing your right leg directly out to the left so it is parallel to the floor, with toes pointing to the wall behind you. If holding your leg out to the side is painful or difficult, place a block or folded blanket under your right foot to support it.

To come out, return to version 1 by bringing your leg back to vertical. Then use the steps for coming out of version 1.

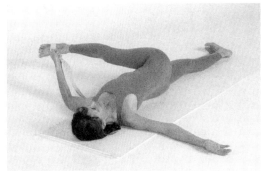

4

RECLINED TWIST (*Jathara Parivartanasana*)

This mildly stimulating pose improves your ability to twist while strengthening and stretching the muscles of your back and abdomen. We prescribe this pose for mild lower back pain, fatigue, preparing for other twists, and as a counter pose for forward bends and backbends.

CAUTIONS: If you have been told to avoid deep twists, or have lower back pain, sacroiliac problems, osteoporosis, or lumbar spine arthritis, try version 2 or 4 or skip this pose.

Version 1: Classic Pose

Start in version 4 of Relaxation Pose. Bring your knees in toward your chest until your thighs are vertical and your shins are parallel with the floor. Stretch your arms out to your sides, with the palms of your hands facing up. Drop your legs and hips gently to the floor to your right so your outer right hip and leg are resting on the floor. Keep the ends of your knees even with each other. If you feel pinching in the back of your left shoulder, lift your left shoulder blade and arm a few inches off the floor and reach your left arm toward the left side of the mat.

To come out, swing your legs back up to center and lower down to the starting position.

Version 2: Gentle Twist

This is a milder version for those who need a gentle alternative or to use as a warm-up for more challenging twists.

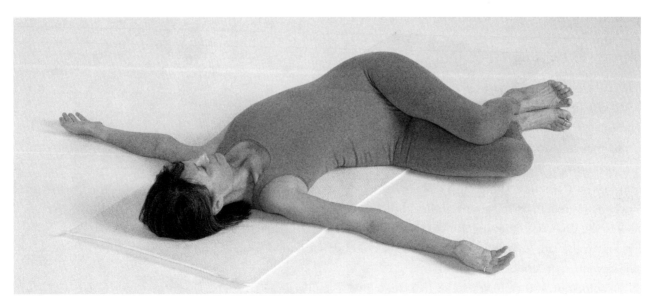

1

Start in version 4 of Relaxation Pose with your feet several inches apart. Then drop your legs to the right, so your outer right leg rests on the floor or is as close to it as possible. Allow your feet to stay apart so your knees do not stack up. Keep your shoulder blades even on the floor. If comfortable, gently turn your head in the opposite direction of your legs.

To come out, swing your legs back to the starting position.

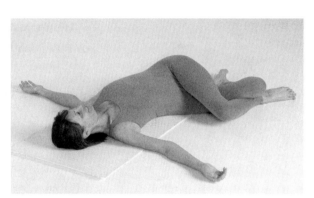

2

Version 3: Crossed Knees

This is a more challenging option that increases the outer hip stretch and builds more core strength.

Start in version 4 of Relaxation Pose. Cross your left thigh tightly over your right. Then, keeping your right foot on the floor, shift your hips an inch or two to the left. Tip both knees up and in toward your chest and take your arms out to your sides, with palms facing up. From there, follow the directions for the classic pose, allowing your legs to drop to the right and come to the floor. If your left shoulder blade cannot stay on the floor, allow it (and your arm) to float.

To come out, swing your legs back toward center and bring your right foot back to the floor. Then uncross your legs and move your hips back to center before changing the cross of your legs and repeating on the other side.

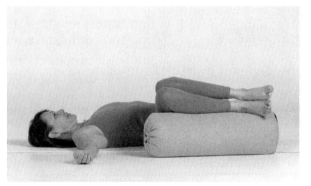

3

Version 4: Restorative Twist

This is a gentle alternative for those who want a mild twist or an option for a more restorative experience.

Start in version 4 of Relaxation Pose, with a bolster on the right side of your mat, parallel with the long edge. Set up as for the classic pose, with your arms out to your sides and your legs tipped in, ready to drop to your right. Release both legs to the right and rest your lower right leg and knee on the bolster. Broaden your chest and relax your shoulder blades onto the floor. Close your eyes if desired.

To come out, gently swing your legs back to center and return your feet to the floor.

4

RELAXATION POSE (*Savasana*)

This powerful resting pose provides deep physical relaxation, allowing you to completely relax your musculoskeletal system in an anatomically neutral position. It also triggers the relaxation response if you practice it with a mental focus. We prescribe this pose for physical tension, lower back pain, stress, fatigue, insomnia, and quieting the mind.

CAUTIONS: Those with lower back pain should try version 3 or 4 and work toward version 1. Those with symptomatic hiatal hernia, acid reflux, sinus congestion, or allergy drainage may not be able to lie flat, so try keeping your hips on the floor but add a prop under your torso and head or skip the pose entirely. If lying on your back causes anxiety, try a prone position, such as Child's Pose.

Version 1: Classic Pose

This version is only for people who are comfortable with no support and can keep their heads in a neutral position. Others should do version 2, 3, or 4.

Lie on your back with your knees bent. Straighten your legs and position them eight to ten inches apart. Turn your arms out so your palms face up and your hands are six to eight inches from your body. Position your head evenly between your shoulders and facing straight up toward the ceiling (not turning to one side). Adjust your body so it's as symmetrical as possible, and your weight is evenly distributed. Make a commitment to staying still and turn your awareness inward.

To come out, move slowly. Bend your knees, placing the soles of your feet on the floor. Then turn over onto your right side. Use your hands to push yourself up to a seated position, allowing your head to release downward until you are upright.

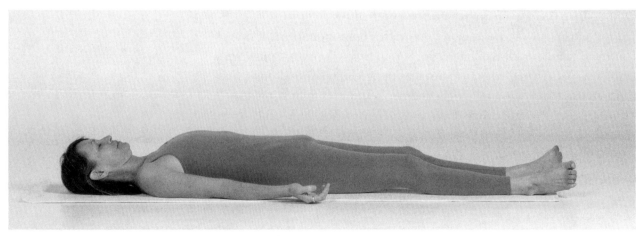

1

Version 2: Head Support

This alternative is for those who need support to keep their heads in a neutral position and for those with head forward syndrome or neck pain. You can include this head support for any other version of Relaxation Pose, as well as any other reclined pose.

Place a folded blanket near the end of your mat where your head will be. (Experiment with its thickness to find the height that suits you best.) When you come into the pose, rest only your head on the blanket (not your neck), with your shoulders resting comfortably on the floor. Use the steps in the classic pose for aligning yourself.

To come out, use the steps for the classic pose.

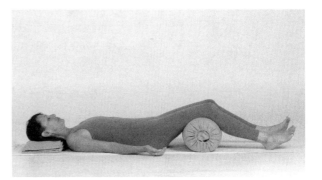

2

Version 3: Legs over Bolster

This alternative is for those with lower back discomfort when lying flat on the floor. It's also a good counter pose for backbends, twists, or forward bends.

Place a bolster crosswise on your mat where you estimate your knees will be and add a support for your head if desired. Lie on your back, with your buttocks on the floor in front of the bolster and the backs of your knees on top of the bolster. Use the steps in the classic pose for aligning yourself, moving the bolster if needed to comfortably support your legs.

To come out, use the steps for the classic pose.

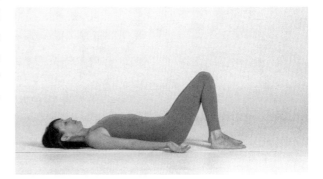

3

Version 4: Constructive Rest

4

This is an alternative for those who experience discomfort lying flat on the floor. It's also a good option for resting your back.

Lie on your back with your knees bent and the soles of your feet on the floor. Position your feet so they are hip-distance apart and far enough away from your sitting bones so your shins are either perpendicular to the floor or slanting away from your pelvis. Let your knees fall toward each other, so the back of your pelvis widens. To allow complete relaxation, you could loosely tie your legs together with a strap just above your knees.

To come out, use the steps for the classic pose, starting by rolling onto your side.

SAGE'S TWIST 3 (*Marichyasana 3*)

This stimulating, challenging twist helps to improve your twisting ability while strengthening your spinal bones and strengthening and stretching your abdominal, chest, and back muscles along with your outer hips, hamstrings, and inner thighs. We prescribe this pose for posture, spine health, fatigue, stimulating digestion, and as a counter pose for backbends and forward bends.

CAUTIONS: For those with lower back pain, herniated discs, or sacroiliac problems, if the pose worsens pain, skip it. Those with osteoporosis and pregnant women in the last two trimesters should do open twists instead, such as version 4 of Easy Sitting Twist. If you feel knee pain in the bent leg, try moving that foot a few inches forward.

Version 1: Classic Pose

Sit tall, with legs extended forward and hands by your hips. Bend your right knee and place your right foot near your right sitting bone, a few inches to the side of the straight leg. Place your right hand on the floor behind your right hip and reach your left arm up toward the ceiling. Turn your upper belly and chest toward your right leg as you bend your left elbow and bring it across the outside of your right knee, pressing it back into your outer knee and leg. Keep your head in a neutral position or turn to face your right shoulder.

To come out, release the twist, place your hands on the floor, and straighten your right leg to come back to the starting position.

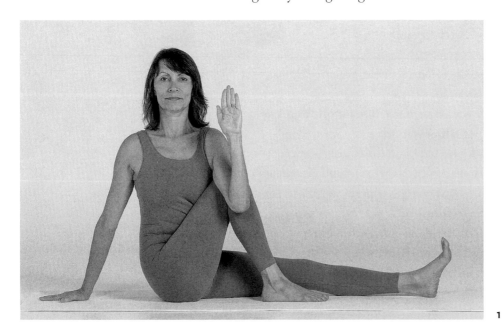

1

Version 2: Hand on Knee

This alternative is for those who can't bring their elbow to the outside of the knee. It is even more accessible if you also sit on a folded blanket as in version 3.

To come into the pose, follow the steps for the classic pose. When you bend your left elbow, hook your left hand around the front of your right knee as you come into the twist.

To come out, use the steps for the classic pose.

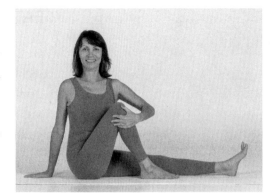

2

Version 3: Seated on Prop

This is an alternative for those with tight hamstrings or stiff or rounded lower backs.

Fold a blanket into a narrow rectangle and place it crosswise on your mat. Sit on the thicker folded edge of the blanket and come into the starting position. From there, follow the steps for the classic pose, using the arm position for either the classic pose or version 2. If you can't place your right hand on the floor without leaning back, use a block to support it so your spine remains vertical and upright.

To come out, use the steps for the classic pose.

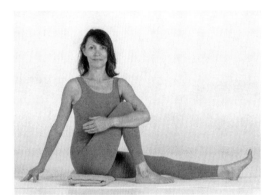

3

Version 4: Foot Crossed over Leg

This challenging option is for those with fairly open outer hips.

Take the starting position for the classic pose. Bend your right leg and bring your right foot toward your right sitting bone. Then step your right foot up and over your left leg and place the sole of your foot on the floor, to the outside of the middle of your left thigh. If your foot cannot easily remain flat on the floor or if your right sitting bone lifts way off the floor, return to versions 1–3 for now. From here, use the steps for the classic pose to move into the twist.

To come out, release the twist and step your right foot back over your left leg. Then use the steps for the classic pose.

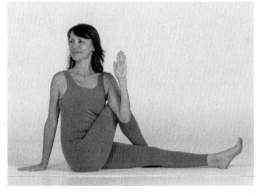

4

SEATED FORWARD BEND (*Paschimottanasana*)

This quieting pose stretches the muscles and fascia of your entire back body, from your heels to the back of your head. For some, folding inward is soothing to the nervous system and quieting for the mind and emotions. We prescribe this pose for stress, anxiety, insomnia, and stimulating digestion.

CAUTIONS: Those with lower back pain, herniated discs, torn hamstring tendons, or sacroiliac problems should try version 2, 3, or 4 or skip this pose if it worsens symptoms. Those with osteoporosis should only do version 2 or 4, and those with wedge fractures should only do version 2. Pregnant women in the last two trimesters should practice only version 4. If any version worsens the symptoms of depression, don't practice it.

Version 1: Classic Pose

Unless you are very flexible, add a support under your hips and keep a strap handy. Sit with your legs straight out in front of you, ankles and feet bent to 45 degrees or flexed to 90 degrees. With an extended spine, reach your arms overhead and tip forward from your hips. When your hips stop rotating, reach your hands toward your feet, wrapping either your fingers or a strap around them. Then mindfully release into the forward bend, without pulling your chest closer to your thighs. Back off if the stretch is too intense.

To come out, engage your leg muscles, release your hands, and swing to an upright position, with your arms reaching above your head. Then release your arms.

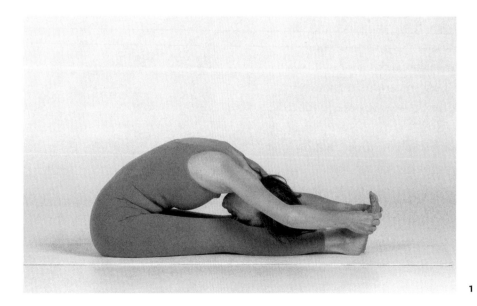

1

Version 2: Straight Back (Extended Spine)

This alternative is for those who cannot safely round their spines and those with very tight legs and hips.

Set up as for the classic pose with a folded blanket under your pelvis and a strap, and follow the initial steps for entering the pose. After tipping from your hips and bringing your hands into position, instead of rounding your spine forward, keep your spine extended as if trying to do a slight backbend. Align your head and neck with your spine (don't tip your head back). Back off if the stretch is too intense.

To come out, use the steps for the classic pose.

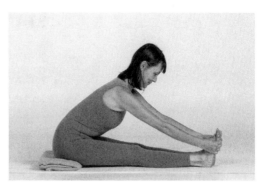

2

Version 3: Bolster under Knees

This alternative is helpful for those who are very tight in the hamstrings and buttocks. It's also an option for a more relaxing experience.

Before coming into the pose, place a round bolster or a thick blanket roll crosswise underneath your knees, so your knees are bent, relaxed, and completely supported. From there, use the steps for the classic pose. Look for a reasonable stretch sensation along the backs of your legs and spine.

To come out, use the steps for the classic pose.

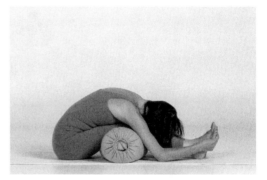

3

Version 4: Head and Arms on Chair

This option provides a more restorative experience and is an alternative for those who cannot safely round their spines or who have tight hips and legs.

Place one folded blanket (more if you are taller) on the chair seat and another on the mat in front of the chair, far enough away so you can take the final pose with a straight or only slightly rounded spine. Then sit on the edge of the blanket, extending your legs between the chair legs. Use the steps for coming into the classic pose, placing your forearms on the seat, and resting your head on your arms, gently rounding your spine only if necessary.

To come out, slowly roll up to a sitting position. Then bend your knees a bit and use your hands to help you scoot away from the chair.

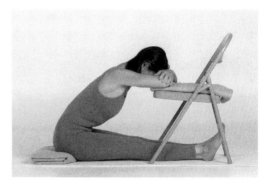

4

STANDING FORWARD BEND (*Uttanasana*)

This quieting pose stretches the muscles and fascia along the entire back surface of your body, including your legs, buttocks, back, and neck. We prescribe this pose for circulation, stress, anxiety, warming up for standing and seated poses, and as a resting pose between standing poses.

CAUTIONS: For those with lower back pain, torn hamstring tendons, or herniated lumbar discs, try version 2, skip this pose, or practice Half Downward-Facing Dog Pose instead. Those with nasal congestion or sinus pressure should do Half Downward-Facing Dog Pose.

Version 1: Classic Pose

Start in Mountain Pose with your feet about hip-distance apart and your hands on your hips. Tip forward from your hip joints, keeping your spine in neutral alignment as long as you can. When you feel your pelvis bones no longer roll forward over your upper thighbones, allow your spine to gently round forward and down until you reach a comfortable stretch. Place your hands or fingertips next to or in front of your feet, or, if they can't reach the floor, place blocks under your hands or bend your elbows and clasp opposite arms. Keep your arms and the sides of your torso strong and active.

To come out, with strong legs, swing up to standing with a straight spine, arms either out to the sides or forward.

Version 2: Bent Knees

This is an alternative for beginners and those with chronic tightness in the back body, including hamstrings, buttocks, or lower back.

Start in Mountain Pose. Bend your knees a few inches and keep them bent as you tip forward from your hip joints and follow the steps for coming into the classic pose.

To come out, still keeping your knees slightly bent, swing up to standing with your spine straight and your arms out to your sides.

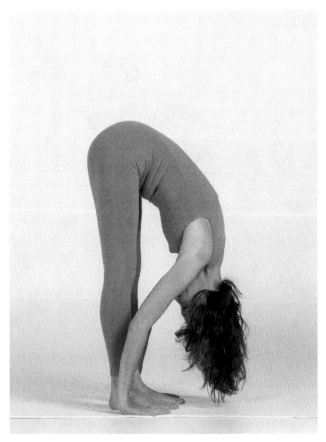

1

Version 3: Block between Thighs

This option strengthens your inner thigh muscles, and squeezing the block as you come out of the pose can make the movement less stressful for lower back muscles.

In Mountain Pose, place a block on either its narrow or middle width between your midthighs, adjusting your feet so you can easily squeeze the block firmly. Slightly rotate your inner thighs toward each other, as if you were going to roll the block slightly backward. From here, follow the steps for the classic pose and maintain your squeeze on the block through the entire pose.

To come out, squeeze the block with your legs as you use the steps for the classic pose.

Version 4: Head and Arm Support

This is an option for a more restorative experience that is very quieting for your nervous system.

Start by facing a chair, with the seat about one foot in front of you. If the seat is hard, place a folded blanket or towel on it. Follow the steps for coming into the classic pose, but place your forearms on the chair seat and rest your head on your stacked hands. Those who are tight may need to bend your knees slightly. If your head doesn't easily come down to meet your hands, add another prop to raise your arms up. Keep your legs somewhat active while releasing from your hips to your head onto the support of the chair.

To come out, engage your legs, bend your knees slightly, and roll up slowly to Mountain Pose.

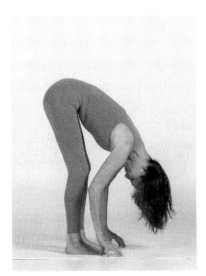

2

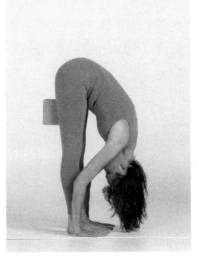

3

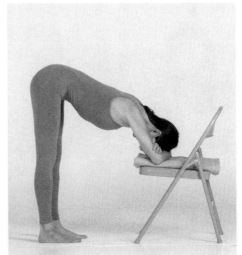

4

SIDE PLANK POSE (*Vasisthasana*)

This challenging arm balance builds strength and stability in your arms, shoulders, and core while improving your balance in an unusual orientation. We prescribe this pose for bone strength in wrists and spine, concentration, and cultivating equanimity.

CAUTIONS: Those with wrist pain should approach this pose cautiously, starting with version 2 or 4. Those with shoulder pain or a history of shoulder joint dislocation should practice version 4 until they are ready for the classic version. Because looking up toward the top arm can create neck pain, we recommend looking forward or down in versions 1–3. Those with newly diagnosed or poorly controlled high blood pressure should hold the pose for only four breaths.

Version 1: Classic Pose

From Downward-Facing Dog Pose, come into a modified Plank Pose, with your shoulders just behind the line of your hands so your hips are a bit high. Shift your weight onto your right arm and rotate your chest and hips up toward the left, with the edges of your feet touching the floor.

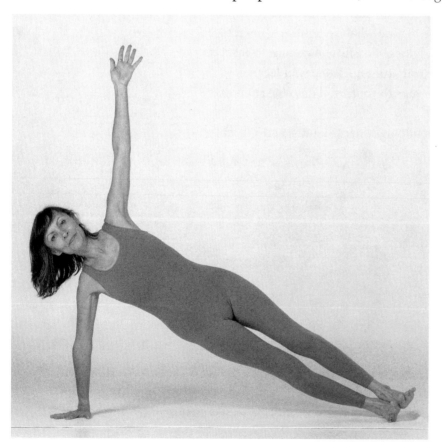

Bring your left hand onto your left hip and stack the inner edge of your left foot on the inner edge of your right foot. Align your legs, hips, torso, and head in a diagonal line and bring your left arm above your left shoulder so it aligns with your right arm. Either look forward or down at your bottom hand.

To come out, separate your stacked feet and return to modified Plank Pose and then Downward-Facing Dog Pose. Drop into Child's Pose to rest and release your right wrist and hand.

Version 2: Foot in Front

This alternative is for those who find it difficult to balance in the classic pose.

Come into modified Plank Pose as described above. Then as you shift your weight onto your right arm, tip both heels to the right until the edges of your feet touch the floor. Keep the left foot, which is on its inner edge, where it is in front of your right foot. (Some people with more flexible feet and ankles can bring the sole of the front foot flat on the floor.) From here, use the steps for the classic pose.

To come out, use the steps for the classic pose.

Version 3: Forearm Version

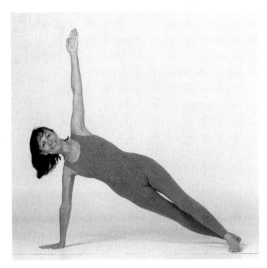

2

This alternative is for those with wrist or hand problems.

Start in version 4 of Downward-Facing Dog Pose, forearms on the floor. Come into a modified Plank Pose with your shoulders over your elbows. Then bring your right forearm 90 degrees to the left so it is perpendicular to your body, right shoulder over right elbow. From there, move into the pose and align your hips, chest, and head as in the classic version. You can either stack your feet as in the classic pose or keep them separated as in version 2. Press down firmly with your entire right forearm to evenly distribute your weight on it. Reach your top arm up and position your head as in the classic pose.

To come out, separate your stacked feet and swivel your forearms parallel to come into the modified Plank Pose. Then return to version 4 of Downward-Facing Dog Pose.

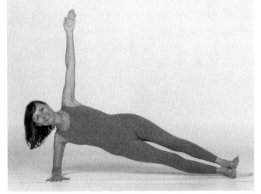

3

Version 4: Hand on Wall

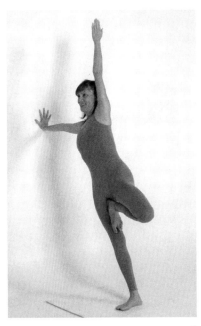

This alternative is for those who are not ready for the full pose and those who can't get down to and up from the floor. It's also a good warm-up for the classic pose.

Stand with your right side to a wall, close enough so you can reach your right arm out to your side, parallel with the floor, and place your palm flat on the wall with fingers pointing up. Step both feet out away from the wall until your right foot is positioned directly under your left shoulder, with your left foot next to your right foot. Check that you are standing at an angle now, with some of your weight being supported by your hand on the wall. Bend your left knee and bring your left foot into Tree Pose position. Then bring your left arm up and alongside your left ear.

To come out, lower your left arm and leg. Then walk your feet a bit closer to the wall into Mountain Pose.

4

SUPPORTED BACKBEND

This accessible, mildly stimulating supported pose stretches the muscles and fascia of your front body, lengthwise from belly to chest and sideways from breastbone out to shoulders, while restoring the natural curves of your spine. We prescribe this pose for lower back pain, posture, fatigue, improving breath capacity, preparing for active backbends, and as a counter pose to forward bends and twists.

CAUTIONS: If you feel lower back pain in the pose, bend your knees and place your feet on the floor. Those with neck pain or arthritis should try version 4. If you have a shoulder injury or shoulder pain, try version 2, taking your arms up only as far as you can without pain. People with severe kyphosis (upper back rounding) may need to use a much smaller roll under the chest and lots of head support.

Version 1: Classic Pose

Place a bolster crosswise on your mat, and add a folded blanket for your head if desired. Sit one to two feet in front of the bolster (depending on your height), with knees bent and feet on the floor. Use your hands to guide yourself back and down onto the bolster, arching your spine to bring your head onto the floor. Support your upper back on the bolster, with the lower tips of your shoulder blades in the center. Take your arms out to your sides along the top edge of the bolster, bending them into a cactus position or keeping them straight. Lengthen your legs along the floor, firm your leg muscles, and softly flex your feet.

To come out, bend your knees and place your feet on the floor. Then roll off the props onto your side and slowly come up to sitting.

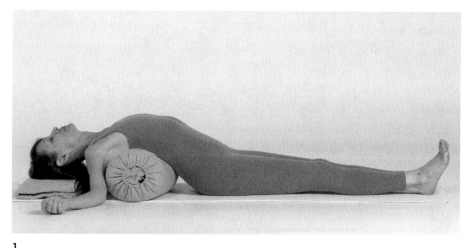

1

Version 2: Arms Overhead

This is an option for greater opening of your spine and front body and for improving shoulder range of motion.

Come into the classic version. If you wish to use a strap on your arms as pictured, place it around your arms so they are shoulder-width apart, then press outward. Next, bring your arms straight up toward the ceiling with your palms facing each other, and actively reach upward. Then slowly bring your arms overhead, reaching for the wall behind you. Press your heels forward as you reach your hands back.

To come out, lift your arms back up toward the ceiling, remove the strap if you're using one, and release your arms down toward the floor. Then use the steps for the classic pose.

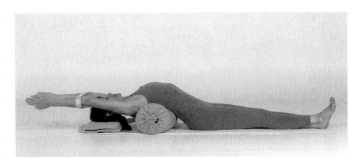

2

Version 3: Block and Head Support

This is an option for greater opening of your upper spine. The blanket under your head is helpful if your neck is uncomfortable when dropping back (the blanket could be used in the first two versions as well).

To set up for the pose, place the block on its lowest height crosswise on the mat, about where the bolster is in the classic pose, and place the folded blanket where your head will be. From here, follow the steps for coming into the classic pose, with the lower tips of your shoulder blades resting on the center of the block. For your head support, experiment to find the right height for you.

To come out, use the steps for the classic pose.

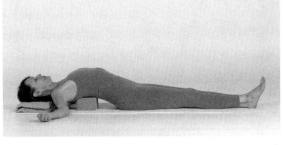

3

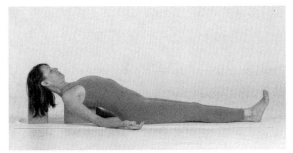

4

Version 4: Using Two Blocks

This option increases spine flexibility and stretches your front body, while eliminating the backbend of your neck and head. It's also an option for a more restorative experience.

To set up for the pose, place the first block on its middle height lengthwise on the mat and place the second block on its highest height about six inches behind the first. Sit one or two feet in front of the first block (depending on your height), with your knees bent and your feet on the floor. Arch your spine and use your hands to guide yourself back and down onto the first block. Position your spine so the first block is between your shoulder blades, and your head is on the second block. (If needed, come out of the pose and move the blocks to better positions.) Take your arms out to the sides and straighten your legs.

To come out, use the steps for the classic pose.

TREE POSE (*Vrksasana*)

This energizing pose strengthens and stretches your upper and lower body and strengthens the core muscles at the sides of your torso as it improves your balance. We prescribe this pose for posture, stiffness in the hips, upper back, and shoulders, concentration, and cultivating equanimity.

CAUTIONS: Avoid placing the heel of your raised foot against the inside of the knee joint; it should always be either above or below it. If you have poor balance, start with version 2 or practice with your back to a wall. If you have an acute ankle sprain, wait until the swelling and pain have resolved before trying this pose. If you have a shoulder injury or shoulder pain, take your arms up only as far as you can without pain or do version 4.

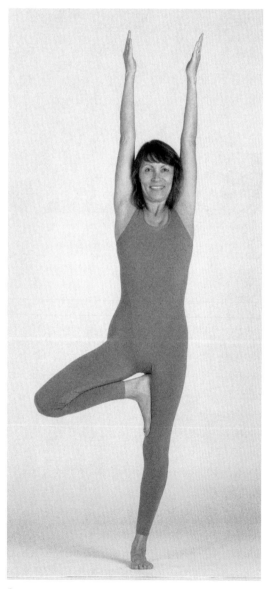

1

Version 1: Classic Pose

Start in Mountain Pose with your feet a few inches apart. Shift your weight onto your left foot and bend your right knee, coming onto the ball of your right foot. Swing your right knee 45 degrees out to the right and place your right foot against your left thigh, with the heel somewhere between your left groin and your midthigh, with toes pointing straight down. Keep your hip points facing forward and the top edge of your pelvis parallel with the floor. Turn your right leg out to a comfortable angle and press your right foot firmly into your left thigh as you firm your left thigh back into your right foot. Bring your arms overhead, in line with your ears if possible, and press down into your standing foot as you lengthen up away from it.

To come out, slowly release your arms and lifted leg back to the starting position.

Version 2: Knee on the Wall

This is an alternative for beginners and those with poor balance or a fear of falling.

Stand perpendicular to a wall with your right hip about one foot away. Shift your weight onto your left foot and bring your right foot into Tree Pose position. Bring your right knee against the wall by using your left foot to heel-toe your body a bit closer to it, while maintaining the hip alignment of the classic pose (check that your left foot is slightly under your pelvis and not directly under your left hip). When your knee is on the wall, bring your arms overhead and work on your foot-thigh squeeze and a rooting-lifting action as in the classic pose.

To come out, bring your right foot down to the floor and your arms down to your sides. Turn to the other direction to do the second side.

Version 3: Foot to Calf

This alternative is for those who cannot easily take the lifted leg position in the classic pose and is a good version for beginners.

Come into the classic pose, placing your right foot against the inner calf muscle of your standing leg. As you balance with arms overhead, press your right foot firmly against your left calf and your left calf against your right foot.

To come out, use the steps for the classic pose.

Version 4: Ball of Foot on Floor

This is an easy alternative for people with balance problems and good for those with a weak or recently sprained ankle.

Start in Mountain Pose. Shift your weight onto your left foot and bend your right knee, coming onto the ball of your right foot. Then slide your right heel up against the inside of your left ankle, so your right heel is just above your left ankle bone but the ball of your foot and your toes are on the ground. Press your right heel firmly into your left ankle and your left ankle back into your right heel. Bring your hands into Prayer position in front of your heart.

To come out, use the steps for the classic pose.

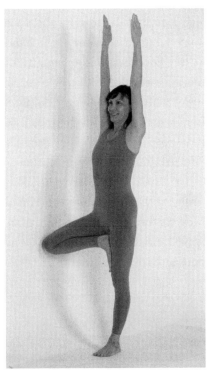

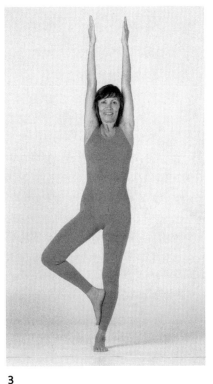

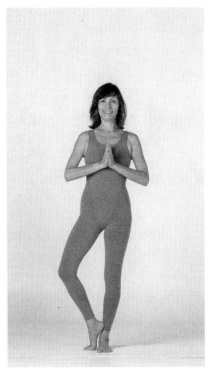

2

3

4

TRIANGLE POSE (*Utthita Trikonasana*)

This energizing pose strengthens and stretches your upper and lower body and strengthens the core muscles at the sides of your torso. We prescribe this pose for fatigue, bone strength in the hips, balance, stiffness in the legs, hips, and shoulders, and as a preparation for other standing poses, forward bends, and twists.

CAUTIONS: If you have lower back pain, torn hamstring tendons, or sacroiliac problems, come up higher if you feel pain or skip the pose entirely. Because looking up toward your top arm can create neck pain, we recommend looking forward or down. If you have a shoulder injury or shoulder pain, take your arms out only as far as you can without pain. Those with newly diagnosed or poorly controlled high blood pressure should hold the pose for only four breaths.

Version 1: Classic Pose

From Mountain Pose, step your feet four to five feet apart. Turn your right foot and leg out 90 degrees, turn your left foot in about 10 degrees, and

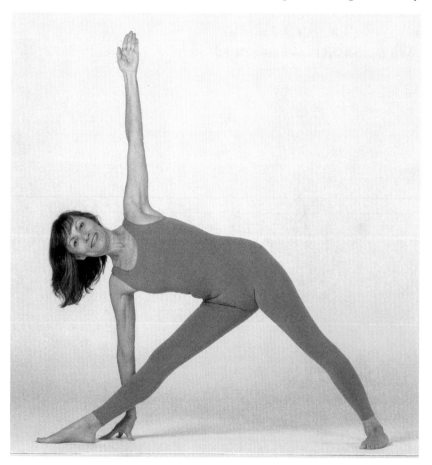

allow your hips to rotate slightly to the right without turning your chest. Raise your arms to be parallel with the floor, then lengthen your torso out over your right leg, tipping your pelvis over your right leg. Keeping both sides of your waist long, bring your right hand to the floor just under your right shoulder and your left arm directly above your left shoulder. Lengthen from your tailbone to the crown of your head and either look straight forward or down at your right foot.

To come out, keep your legs strong and lift your torso and head back to the upright starting position. Release your arms to your sides and turn your feet to parallel.

1

Version 2: Bottom Hand on Block

This alternative is for those who cannot place a hand on the floor while maintaining a long spine.

Place a block to the right side of your mat so it will be behind your right heel when you step your legs apart (it's okay to move it later if it isn't in the right place). Then use the steps for coming into the classic pose, bringing your palm or fingertips firmly onto the block. Experiment to find the height of the block that works best for you and allows both sides of your waist and your spine to stay long and parallel.

To come out, use the steps for the classic pose, moving the block to your left side before repeating.

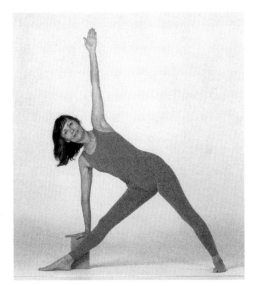

2

Version 3: Top Hand on Waist

This is an alternative for those who have shoulder pain or tightness, tightness in the hips, or balance problems. (If you have trouble balancing in this one, try version 4.)

Take the preparation position for either the classic pose or version 2, but place your left hand on your left hip with your elbow pointing out to the side. Then, when you enter the full pose, keep your left arm in the same position, so your elbow now points directly up. Use the steps for the classic pose for aligning the rest of your body.

To come out, use the steps for the classic pose, leaving your hand on your hip until you come to the upright position and then release both arms.

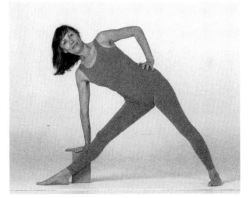

3

Version 4: Bottom Hand on Chair Seat

This alternative is for those who can't bring the bottom hand to a block while maintaining a long spine and is a gentle option for people who have back pain, weakness, or balance problems.

Position a chair so that when you step your feet apart it will be behind your right foot, with the seat facing the long edge of your mat. Then use the steps for coming into the classic pose, bringing your palm or fingertips firmly onto the seat. Because you will be higher up than in the classic pose, your right arm may angle a bit forward and down, so bring your left arm in line with the right.

To come out, use the steps for the classic pose. Then step your feet together into Mountain Pose.

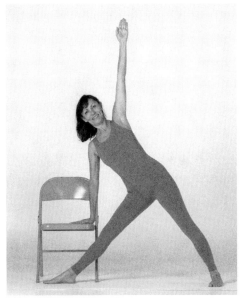

4

UPWARD-FACING DOG POSE
(*Urdhva Mukha Svanasana*)

This energizing and challenging backbend strengthens your arms, chest, shoulders, and legs, improves spinal flexibility, stretches your entire front body, and opens your chest. We prescribe this pose for posture, spine health, bone strength in the wrists and spine, fatigue, and depression.

CAUTIONS: If this pose causes back pain, start with the Cobra and Locust poses instead. Those with wrist and hand pain should modify or skip this pose if it increases pain. Those with abdominal hernias or women with abdominal wall separation should practice this pose with care so it does not worsen your condition or try Bridge Pose instead. If you tend to overarch your lower back, try drawing your front lower ribs back toward your spine to avoid excessive swayback. Those with newly diagnosed or poorly controlled high blood pressure should hold the pose for only four breaths.

Version 1: Classic Pose

Start in Downward-Facing Dog Pose. Shift your shoulders forward into Plank Pose. One at a time, lift your feet and come onto the tops of them, toes pointing back. Pivoting at your shoulders, swing your hips forward toward your wrists, turning your chest forward and up. Keep your shoulders directly over your wrists, press your palms down, firm your arms, and press upward toward your shoulders. Firm your leg muscles, widen your collarbones, and firm your shoulder blades down your back as you keep your chest lifted. Look straight ahead.

To come out, one foot at a time, turn your toes under. Then swing your hips up and back into Downward-Facing Dog Pose. Release your knees to the floor.

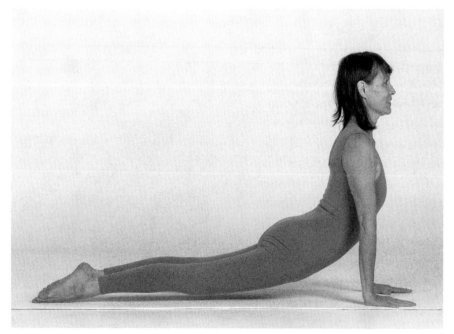

1

Version 2: Toes Turned Under

This is an option for practicing in Sun Salutations or for stretching and strengthening your calves.

Follow the steps for the classic pose but keep your toes turned under. As you come into the backbend, imagine you are pressing your heels into a wall behind you. This will engage your leg muscles to assist your arms in keeping you in the pose. If you feel pain or pinching in your lower back, firm your abdomen back toward your spine.

To come out, use the steps for the classic pose.

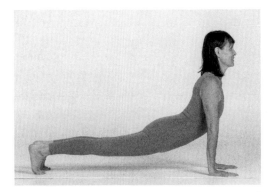

2

Version 3: Hands on Blocks

This alternative is for those who have trouble getting their knees off the floor in the classic pose or who just want a more gradual backbend.

Lie on your belly as you would for Cobra Pose, with two blocks on their lowest height positioned lengthwise next to your middle to lower ribs (move them if needed to ensure your shoulders are directly over your wrists in the pose). With your palms on the blocks, bend your arms like grasshopper legs. Slowly roll your chest and head up, pressing your hands firmly into the blocks as you gradually curl up to straight arms. Press down with the tops of your feet and lift your legs off the floor, keeping your knees straight.

To come out, slowly bend your arms and lower yourself down onto your belly, chest, and chin, taking your arms to your sides.

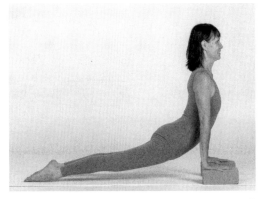

3

Version 4: Using a Chair

This alternative is a good beginner pose to practice before progressing to the classic pose.

Place a chair with its back against a wall. Stand facing the chair about a foot away. Bend your knees and place your hands flat on the chair seat, wrists near the front edge. Then walk your feet away from the chair three to four feet, coming into Downward-Facing Dog Pose on the chair. Shift your shoulders forward over your wrists into Plank Pose. Then swing your hips forward to come into the backbend while pressing back into your heels to firm your legs. Either keep your toes turned under or come onto the tops of your feet.

To come out, swing back into Downward-Facing Dog Pose. Then walk forward and come into Mountain Pose.

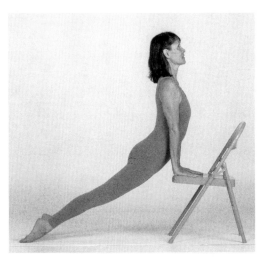

4

UPWARD PLANK POSE (*Purvottanasana*)

This energizing and challenging backbend lengthens the front of your body from your toes to your head, while strengthening your arms, shoulders, and entire back body. We prescribe this pose for posture, bone strength in the wrists and spine, shoulder stiffness, and depression.

CAUTIONS: Those with wrist or hand pain should modify your hand position or try version 4. Those with shoulder pain or a history of dislocation should use caution, possibly staying with version 2. Those with neck pain should keep your head upright or chin tucked to your chest. Those with newly diagnosed or poorly controlled high blood pressure should hold the pose for only four breaths.

Version 1: Classic Pose

Sit with your legs extended, your spine erect over your hips, and your hands on the floor at your sides. Move your hands about six to twelve inches behind your hips, with your palms flat on floor and your fingers pointing forward or any position good for your wrists. Firming your palms down, lengthen through your elbows and lift the lower tip of your breastbone up to bring your chest into a backbend, while keeping your chin and head in a neutral position. Push through your arms and pivot on your heels as you lift your hips up and forward, pressing the balls of your feet forward and down toward the floor. Keep your thighs parallel. Carefully move your head back in line with the arch of your spine, keeping the back of your neck long.

To come out, lower your hips to the floor as you bring your head back to a vertical position. Release your hands and shake out your wrists.

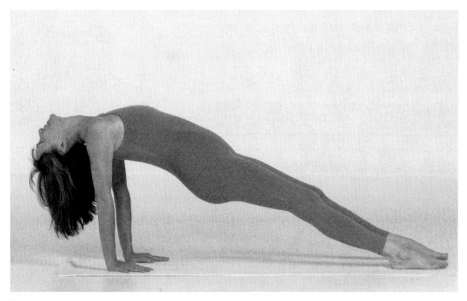

1

Version 2: Seated

This is an alternative for those who are weak or out of shape or those with wrist, shoulder, and neck problems.

Sit with your legs extended, your spine erect over your hips, and your hands on the floor at your sides. Move your hands about six to twelve inches back behind your hips, with your palms flat on the floor. Firm your palms down, lengthen through your elbows, and lift the lower tip of your breastbone up to create a backbend, while keeping your chin and head in a neutral position.

To come out, return to the starting position. Release the tension in your shoulders, neck, and wrists as needed.

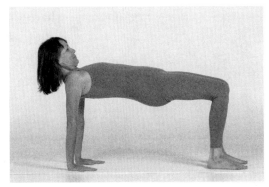

2

Version 3: Reverse Table Pose

This is an easier alternative for those working toward the classic pose and a good option for increasing shoulder flexibility.

Start by coming into version 2. Bend your knees, placing your feet about one-and-a-half feet from your hips. Pressing down into your hands and feet, lift your hips up about six inches and toward your feet a bit, keeping your chin tucked toward your chest. Pressing firmly into your hands and feet, with knees over ankles and shoulders over wrists, gradually lift your hips and chest so your hips line up with your shoulders and knees. Keep your head upright or use the head position for the classic pose.

To come out, lower your hips to the floor. Release the tension in your shoulders, neck, and wrists as needed.

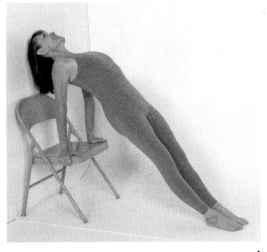

3

Version 4: Using a Chair

This is a gentler alternative for those who lack upper body strength or shoulder flexibility and is a good version for beginners.

Place a chair with its back legs against the wall. Sit on the edge of the seat with your legs together and your knees bent. Place your hands alongside your hips and extend your legs straight out in front of you, with your feet close together. Press your hands into the seat as you lift your hips up, open your chest, and press the balls of your feet into the floor. Align your hips and chest so your body makes a straight line from your feet to your shoulders. If desired, try releasing your head and neck back, maintaining as much length in the back of your neck as possible.

To come out, lower your hips to the seat. Then shake out your wrists and hands.

4

WARRIOR 1 POSE (*Virabhadrasana 1*)

This energizing standing backbend builds strength in your legs, arms, and upper back, while stretching your hips, upper back, and shoulders and challenging your balance. We prescribe this pose for posture, fatigue, bone strength in hips and spine, depression, and as a preparation for other backbends.

CAUTIONS: Those with knee pain should stand with feet closer together, bending your knees less if necessary. Those with lower back pain or sacroiliac problems should shorten their stance about six to twelve inches and, after turning sideways, step each foot a bit out to the side. If you have a shoulder injury or shoulder pain, take your arms up carefully, only going as far as you can without pain. Those with newly diagnosed or poorly controlled high blood pressure should hold the pose for only four breaths.

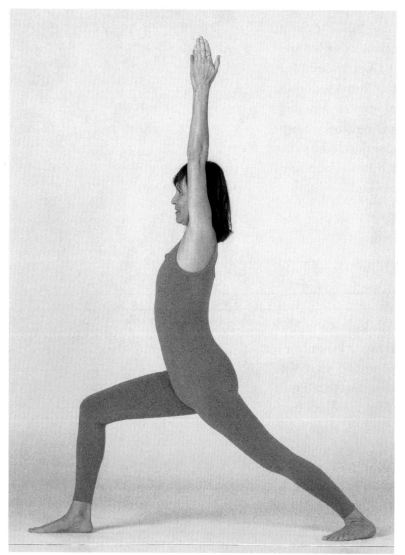

Version 1: Classic Pose

From Mountain Pose, step your feet about three to four feet apart. Turn your right foot and leg out 90 degrees, then pivot your left heel back about four to five inches to turn your left foot and leg in about 45–60 degrees. Rotate your chest and belly toward your right leg. Swing your arms forward and up along the sides of your head, with your palms facing each other, and bend your right knee directly over your right ankle (to no more 90 degrees). Firm the muscles around your left knee to keep your left leg straight and lengthen from your back heel up through your hips, spine, and arms as you arch into a gentle backbend. Balance your head over your shoulders and gaze straight ahead.

To come out, straighten your front leg and release your arms to your sides. Then pivot back to the starting position with feet parallel and wide apart.

1

Version 2: Bird-Wing Arms

This alternative is for those who cannot easily take their arms overhead and a good option for opening the front of the chest.

Follow the steps for the classic pose, but instead of bringing your arms overhead, bend your elbows to 90 degrees and take your arms out to your sides in a bird-wing position. Keep your elbows in line with or slightly below your shoulders and your forearms and hands pointing straight up. Widen your front chest as you relax your shoulders downward. Follow the leg, hip, spine, and head instructions for the classic pose, lengthening up from your back heel to the crown of your head.

To come out, use the steps for the classic pose.

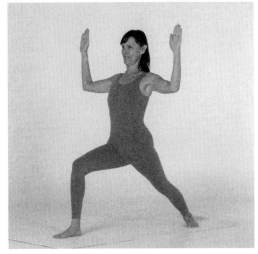

2

Version 3: Hands on Hips

This is an alternative for those with shoulder or balance problems.

Follow the steps for the classic pose, but instead of bringing your arms overhead, bring your hands to your hips. Widen your front chest, move your elbows back a bit, and relax your shoulders downward. Follow the leg, hip, spine, and head instructions for the classic pose, lengthening up from your back heel to the crown of your head.

To come out, use the steps for the classic pose, relaxing your arms by your sides.

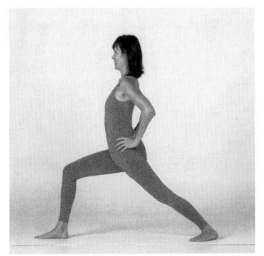

3

Version 4: Hands on Chair Back

This alternative is for those with poor balance or who are not yet strong enough to do the classic pose.

Start in Mountain Pose, a few inches away from the back of a chair, with your hands resting on top of the chair. Step your left foot straight back two and a half to three feet and turn your left foot out about 45 degrees. Then bend your right knee over your ankle. Follow the leg, hip, spine, and head instructions for the classic pose, lengthening up from your back heel to the crown of your head. Press your hands down onto the top of the chair, while keeping your arms long and straight.

To come out, step your left foot forward to match your right foot and straighten both legs. Then come into Mountain Pose with your arms at your sides.

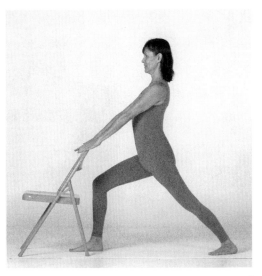

4

WARRIOR 2 POSE (*Virabhadrasana 2*)

This grounding pose strengthens your lower and upper body while stretching your hips, legs, and chest and challenging your balance. We prescribe this pose for posture, fatigue, bone strength in hips, anxiety and depression, and as a preparation for other standing poses.

CAUTIONS: If you have knee problems, don't bend your front knee deeply. If you have a shoulder injury or shoulder pain, take your arms up only as far as you can without pain. Those with newly diagnosed or poorly controlled high blood pressure should hold the pose for only four breaths.

Version 1: Classic Pose

From Mountain Pose, step your feet about four to five feet apart. Turn your right foot and leg out 90 degrees, turn your back foot in about 10 degrees, and allow your hips to rotate slightly to the right without turning your chest. Bring your arms out to your sides, parallel with your shoulders, shoulder blades relaxing down. Bend your right knee directly over your right ankle, up to 90 degrees, with your right knee in line with your middle toe. With hips slightly rotating toward your right foot, rotate your chest toward the long edge of your mat and widen your arms away from each other. If it's comfortable, turn your head to gaze over your right hand.

To come out, straighten your right leg, then turn your feet parallel and relax your arms to your sides.

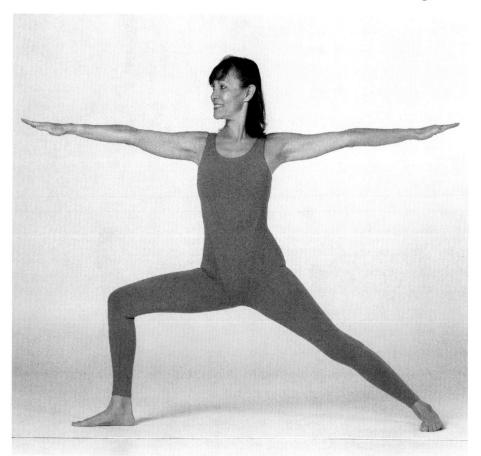

Version 2: Hands on Hips, Feet Closer

This is an easier alternative for beginners and those with tight inner thighs, shoulder problems, or poor balance.

From Mountain Pose, step your feet only about three to four feet apart. Then adjust your legs and feet as in classic pose. Place your hands on your hips, with your elbows away from each other and your shoulder blades relaxing down. Bend your right knee and from here use the alignment instructions for the classic pose for hips, front knee, chest, and head.

To come out, straighten your right leg, then turn your feet parallel and relax your arms to your sides.

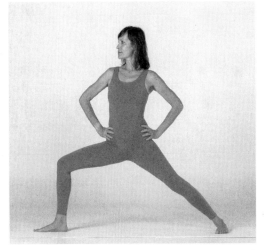

2

Version 3: Using a Chair

This is an alternative for those with balance problems, weakness, or injuries that affect your ability to stand.

Sit on the front edge of a chair (place a folded blanket on the seat if you are tall). Swivel to your right, bringing your right sitting bone and thigh along the seat's front edge and your left sitting bone slightly off the seat. Bend your right knee so it's directly above your ankle, with your foot turned out 90 degrees. Slide your left leg back away from the right until you can straighten your left knee with your left foot on the floor. (Your left leg may need to be forward a few inches.) From here, use the alignment instructions for the classic pose for hips, chest, and head.

To come out, lower your arms, then bend your left knee and swing both legs forward so you sit evenly on the seat's front edge.

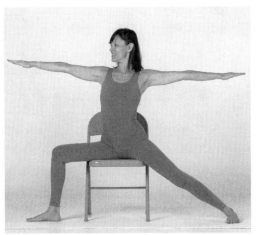

3

Version 4: Reverse Warrior

This challenging option stretches the sides of your chest and arms while improving your balance.

Start in the classic pose. Keeping your front knee aligned with your ankle, bring your right arm up toward the ceiling as you reach your left hand down toward your outer thigh. Keeping your right knee firm, slowly slide your left hand farther down your leg as you side bend your torso over your left leg and reach your right arm up and to the left. Stop when you feel a significant stretch. Either gaze straight ahead or up toward your top hand.

To come out, tip back to the classic pose and then come out as usual.

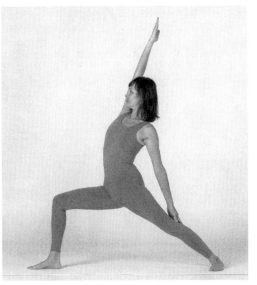

4

WARRIOR 3 POSE (*Virabhadrasana 3*)

This challenging and energizing balance pose strengthens all the muscles along the back of your body, including your buttocks, backs of thighs, and all the back muscles out into your arms, while also stretching your legs, hips, front body, and shoulders and improving your balance. We prescribe this pose for bone strength in hips and spine, concentration, cultivating equanimity, and preparing for backbends.

CAUTIONS: Those with back pain or torn hamstring tendons, try version 4 or bend your bottom knee. For shoulder injury or pain, take arms up only as far as you can without pain or do version 3. For acute ankle sprain, wait until swelling and pain resolve. Those with newly diagnosed or poorly controlled high blood pressure should hold the pose for only four breaths.

Version 1: Classic Pose

Come into the classic version of Warrior 1 Pose. From there, pivot onto the ball of your left foot and tip your torso forward about 45 degrees. Shift your weight onto your right foot and straighten your right leg as you slowly lift your left leg up behind you, tipping your torso and arms forward, parallel with the floor. Focus on keeping your hips even with the floor and reach your arms straight forward, with your head slightly lifted or aligned with your spine and your gaze slightly forward.

To come out, bend your right knee slightly and bring your left foot down into Warrior 1 Pose. From there, release your arms to your sides, straighten your front leg, and pivot to standing with feet parallel and wide apart.

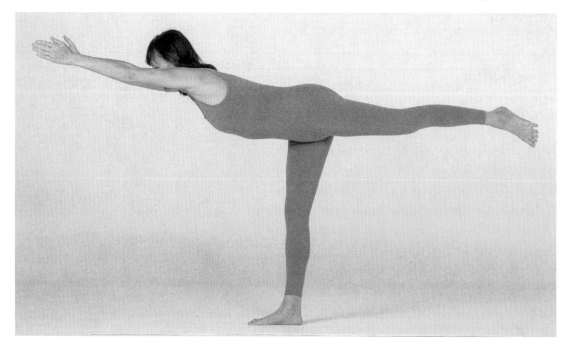

1

Version 2: Using the Wall

This is an easy alternative for beginners or for those who are weak, have balance problems, or are afraid of the classic pose. It's also a good warm-up for other versions.

Come into the classic version of Half Downward-Facing Dog Pose. From there, step your right foot toward your left foot and allow your hips to shift a little to the right so more of your weight is on your right foot. Keeping your hips parallel with the floor, swing your left leg up and back, in line with your arms and torso.

To come out, lower your left foot to the floor, returning to Half Downward-Facing Dog Pose. Then bend your knees, slowly walk forward to standing upright, and shake out your wrists.

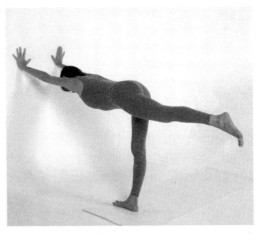

2

Version 3: Arms Back

This alternative is for those who have shoulder problems and those who aren't strong enough for the classic pose. It's also a good option for beginners.

Start in Warrior 1 Pose with arms by your sides. From there, pivot onto the ball of your left foot and tip your torso forward about 45 degrees. Keeping your arms by your sides, shift your weight onto your right foot and straighten your right leg as you slowly lift your left leg and bring your torso parallel with the floor.

To come out, bend your right knee slightly and bring your left foot back and down to the floor into the starting position. From there, straighten your front leg and pivot back to standing with feet parallel and wide apart.

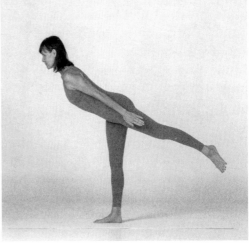

3

Version 4: Tilted Part Way

This alternative is for those who can't come to parallel with the floor and those who want to slowly work their way up to the classic pose. It's also good for beginners.

Start in the classic version of Warrior 1 Pose. From there, pivot onto the ball of your left foot and tip your torso forward about 45 degrees. Shift your weight onto your right foot and straighten your right leg as you slowly lift your left leg up while tipping your torso to an angle that's comfortable for you. Create one long, straight line from your left heel to your fingertips and follow the alignment instructions for the classic pose.

To come out, use the steps for the classic pose.

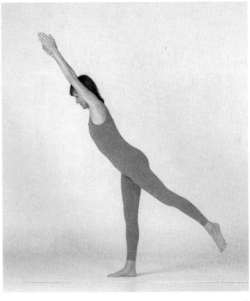

4

DYNAMIC POSES AND FLOW SEQUENCES

In this section, we begin by illustrating the dynamic poses, in which you move in and out of a one pose with your breath. This is followed by illustrations of our flow sequences, in which you link multiple poses together with your breath.

Dynamic Poses

DYNAMIC ARMS OVERHEAD POSE

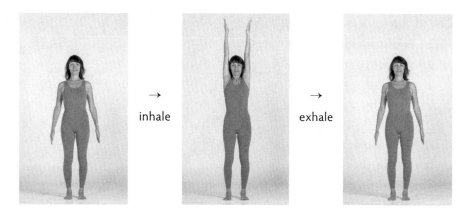

DYNAMIC BRIDGE POSE

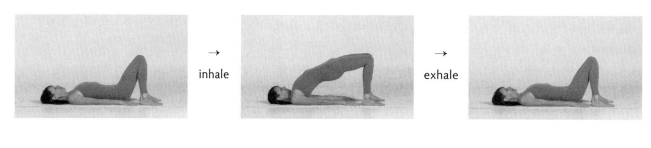

DYNAMIC CAT-COW POSE

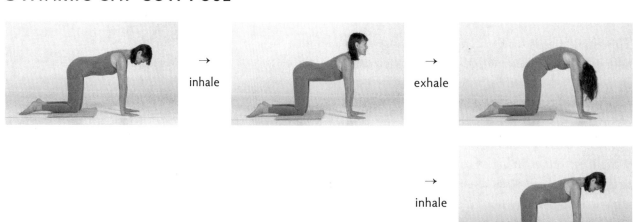

DYNAMIC DOWNWARD-FACING DOG POSE

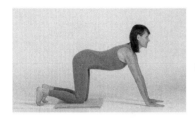 → exhale 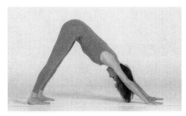 → inhale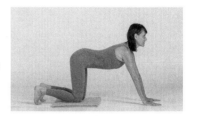

DYNAMIC HUNTING DOG POSE

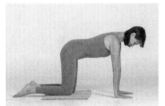 → inhale 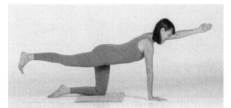 → exhale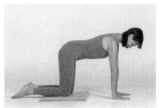

→ inhale 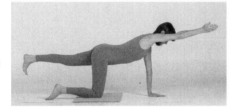 → exhale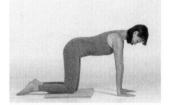

DYNAMIC LOCUST POSE

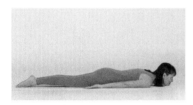 → inhale 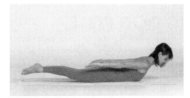 → exhale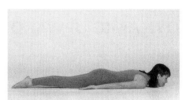

DYNAMIC POWERFUL POSE

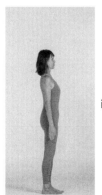 → inhale 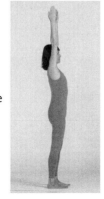 → exhale 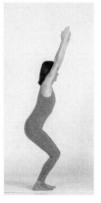 → inhale 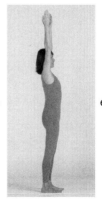 → exhale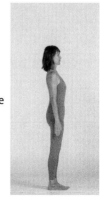

DYNAMIC RECLINED TWIST

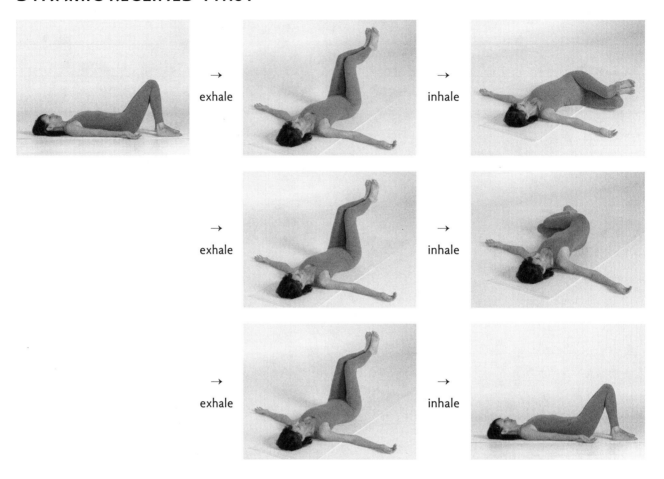

DYNAMIC UPWARD-FACING DOG POSE

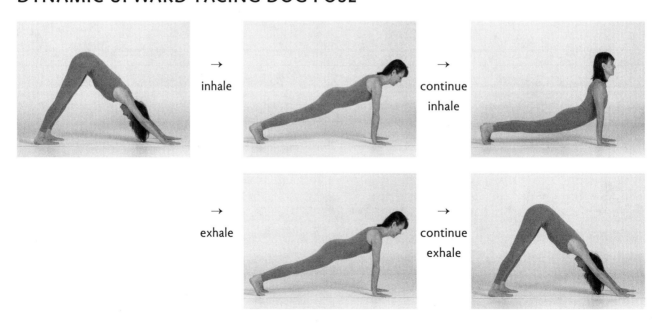

DYNAMIC WARRIOR 1 POSE

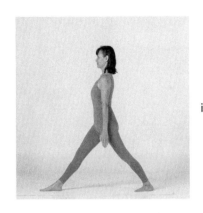 → inhale 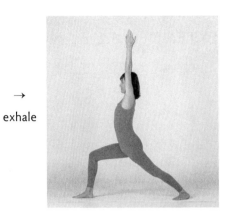 → exhale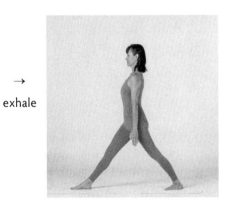

→ inhale 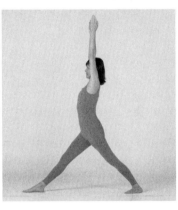 → exhale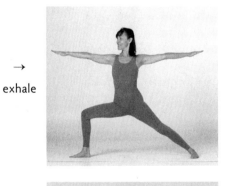

DYNAMIC WARRIOR 2 POSE

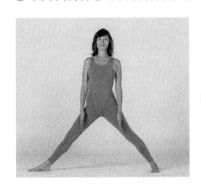 → inhale 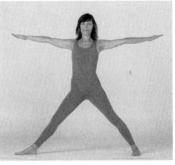 → exhale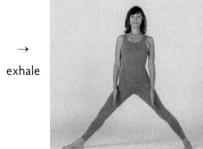

→ inhale 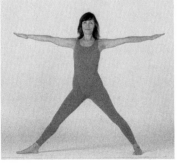 → exhale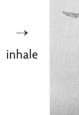

Flow Sequences (Vinyasas)

EXTENDED SIDE ANGLE VINYASA

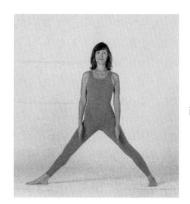 → inhale 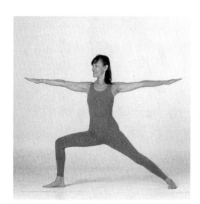 → exhale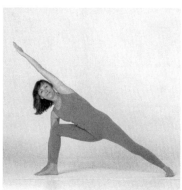

→ inhale 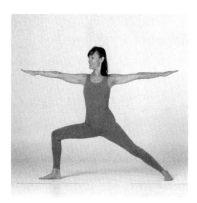 → exhale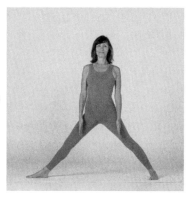

SIDE PLANK VINYASA (ALTERNATE SIDES EVERY OTHER ROUND)

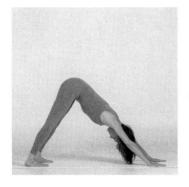 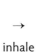 inhale 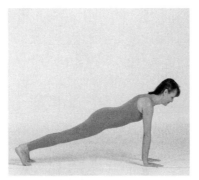 exhale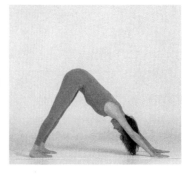

 inhale 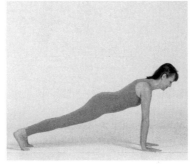  exhale

STANDING FORWARD BEND VINYASA

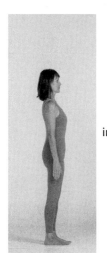 inhale 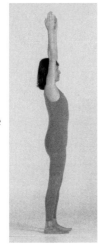 exhale 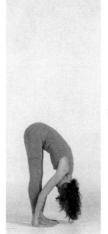 inhale 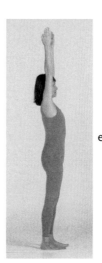 exhale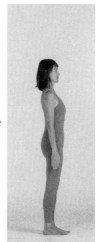

SUN SALUTATION, MINI (ALTERNATE THE LEAD FOOT EVERY OTHER ROUND)

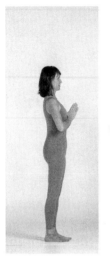 inhale 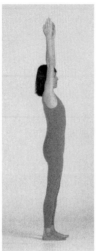 exhale 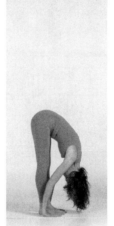 inhale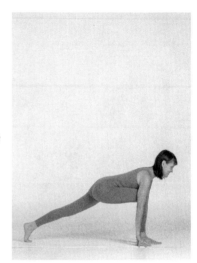

 exhale 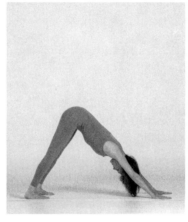 inhale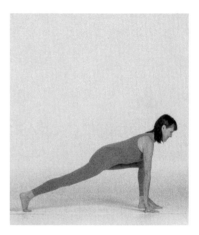

exhale 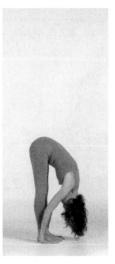 inhale 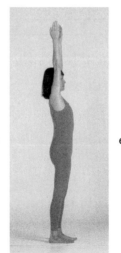 exhale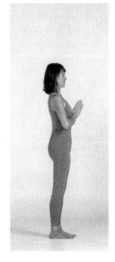

SUN SALUTATION, FULL (ALTERNATE
THE LEAD FOOT EVERY OTHER ROUND)

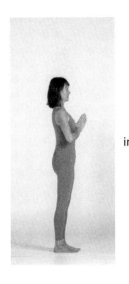

→ inhale

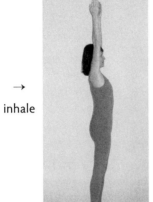

→ exhale

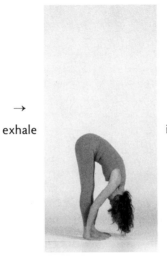

→ inhale

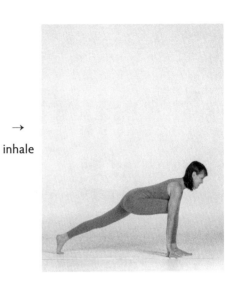

→ exhale

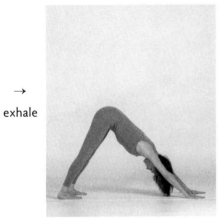

→ inhale

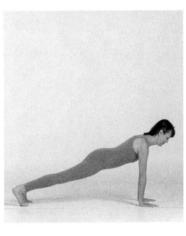

→ inhale (cont.)

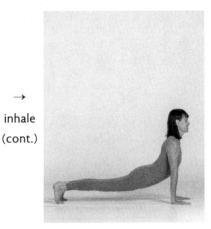

→ exhale

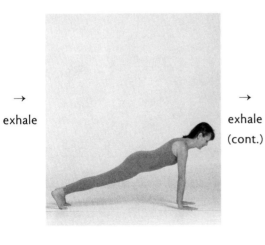

→ exhale (cont.)

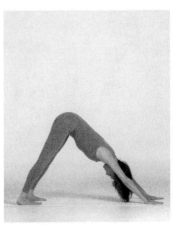

→ inhale

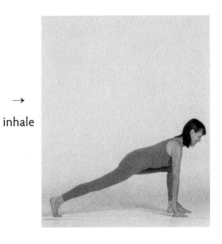

(continued on next page)

→ exhale 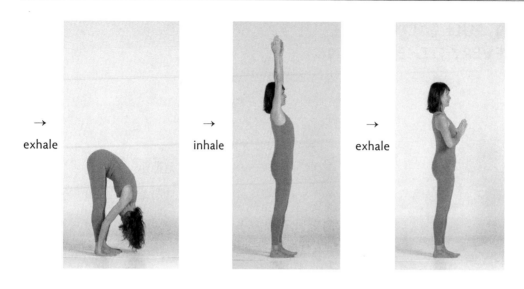 → inhale → exhale

WARRIOR 3 VINYASA

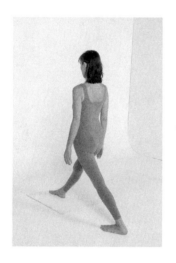 → inhale 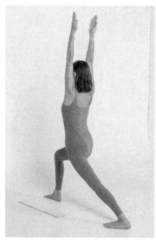 → exhale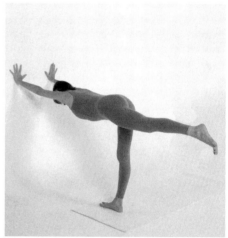

→ inhale 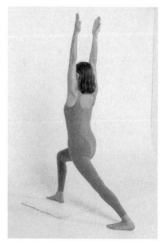 → exhale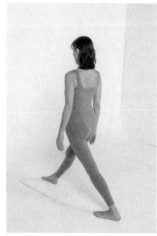

APPENDIX: CONTRAINDICATIONS FOR MEDICAL CONDITIONS

Movements to Avoid Based on Condition

In the table below is a list of medical conditions and the movements that we recommend you avoid for each. If you don't know what a movement type means, see the explanatory tables that follow.

CONDITION	MOVEMENTS TO AVOID
Abdominal pain (such as from irritable bowel syndrome and celiac disease)	Avoid flexion, rotation, and any spinal movement that increases pain.
Acid reflux disease	Avoid flexion of spine and any spinal movement that increases symptoms. Avoid inversions if symptoms worsen.
Anxiety (active symptoms)	Avoid backbends.
Asthma (active symptoms)	Avoid active backbends and use caution with passive backbends.
Back pain, lower	Modify all spinal movements that cause pain and use extra caution for flexion and extension.
Bursitis	Avoid any movement that increases pain or swelling.
Carpal tunnel syndrome (wrist)	Avoid any movement that increases pain or numbness, especially the extension of wrist while weight bearing.
Cataract surgery (recent)	Avoid full inversions.
Degenerative disc disease of spine	Avoid flexion of spine, with or without rotation, and any movement that causes pain.

Diabetes, type 1	Avoid deep spinal twists if insulin is injected into abdomen. Avoid full inversions to avoid risk to eyes. Practice caution with partial or gentle inversions, under guidance of ophthalmologist.
Elbow, golfer's elbow	Avoid flexion of wrist and elbow supination.
Elbow, tennis elbow	Avoid extension of wrist and elbow pronation.
Facet joint arthritis of spine	Avoid extension of spine, with or without rotation, and any movement that causes pain.
Fibromyalgia	Avoid any movement that triggers pain.
Frozen shoulder	Safe to try all movements to your pain tolerance.
Glaucoma	Avoid full inversions.
Hamstring, tear or strain	Avoid flexion of hip.
Headache (active)	Avoid full or partial inversions.
Hernia, groin	Avoid any movement of hip or spine that increases pain or hernia size, especially flexion of hip and spine and adduction of hip.
Hernia, abdominal wall or separation	Avoid extension and flexion of spine.
Herniated discs in lumbar spine	Avoid flexion of spine, with or without rotation, and any movement that causes pain or sciatica.
Hip repair/replacement	Check with surgeon. For some types, avoid internal rotation of hip or flexion of more than 90 degrees.
High blood pressure (hypertension), not controlled	Avoid inversions; deep, sustained spinal rotation and/or flexion; and long holds of standing poses.
Irritable bowel syndrome	Avoid deep spinal twisting or flexion that increases symptoms.
Joint pain with acute or chronic swelling	Avoid any movement that increases pain.
Joint that is hyperflexible	Avoid any movement that goes beyond normal range of motion or causes pain.
Knee pain	Avoid flexion, with or without rotation of knee, and any movement that increases knee pain.
Knee with meniscal tear	Avoid deep flexion, with or without rotation of knee.
Knee with anterior cruciate ligament repair	Avoid deep flexion of knee. Never put spacer (rolled towel or blanket) behind knee in flexion.
Multiple sclerosis	Only gentle movements of joints recommended. Avoid overheating.
Muscle strain	For general muscle strain, avoid movement that stretches the area.
Neck pain (general)	Avoid full inversions. Avoid neck movements that worsen pain.

Numbness in hands or feet	Avoid any movement that causes this.
Obesity	Avoid full inversions.
Osteoarthritis	Avoid any weight-bearing movement at any joint that has painful arthritis. When there is no swelling or only mild pain, attempt to move the joint in all directions if no flare-up of symptoms occurs.
Osteoporosis	Avoid flexion of spine, especially thoracic spine, and use caution with deep rotation of spine.
Peptic ulcers	Avoid any movements that worsen pain, especially deep flexion and rotation of spine.
Pregnancy, second or third trimester	Avoid deep flexion or rotation of spine.
Pubic symphysis separation	Avoid abduction of hips and deep extension of one leg.
Rotator cuff injury	Avoid any movement that causes pinching or pain, especially flexion and extension of shoulder combined with external rotation.
Sacroiliac joint pain or dysfunction	Avoid flexion of spine, with or without rotation of spine, and any movement that increases pain.
Shoulder dislocation history	Avoid any movement that caused shoulder dislocation in past. Check with orthopedic doctor or physical therapist for specific guidelines on those movements.
Shoulder labral tear	Avoid any movement that causes pinching or pain, especially deep flexion, extension, abduction, or adduction, with or without rotation of shoulder.
Scoliosis	Avoid any movement that causes pain (modify with guidance of teacher or yoga therapist). Modify spinal rotation and side bending.
Spinal stenosis	Exercise caution with extension of spine and any movement that increases pain or symptoms.
Spondylolisthesis of spine	Avoid extension of spine and check with orthopedic doctor or physical therapist for additional cautions.
Thoracic outlet syndrome	Avoid full flexion or abduction of shoulder with arms overhead and full inversion handstand and shoulderstand.
Thoracic wedge fractures of spine	Avoid flexion of thoracic spine.
Tingling in hands or feet	Avoid any movement that causes this symptom.
Wrist, ganglion cyst	Depends on location of cyst, but usually avoid any extension of wrist, with or without weight bearing.

Movements of the Hip Joint

MOVEMENT	DESCRIPTION
Flexion	Moving thigh in toward front of lower torso or bringing front of lower torso toward thigh (forward bend of hips). Examples: Lifted leg in Reclined Leg Stretch, tipping pelvis in Standing Forward Bend
Extension	Raising back of thigh toward back of lower torso or bringing back of lower torso toward your leg. Example: Lifted legs in Locust Pose
Abduction	Moving your leg or legs to the side, away from the midline of your body. Example: Stepping feet apart from Mountain Pose to wide stance for Triangle Pose
Adduction	Moving one leg across the other (example: version 3 of Reclined Leg Stretch) or moving a leg that was out to the side back toward the midline of the body (example: stepping back into Mountain Pose from a wide-leg stance)
External rotation	Turning your leg out within your hip socket so the leg turns away from the midline of your body. Example: Turning the front leg out 90 degrees in Triangle Pose
Internal rotation	Turning your leg in within your hip socket so the leg turns toward the midline of your body. Example: Setting up the back leg for Triangle Pose

Movements of the Spine

MOVEMENT	DESCRIPTION
Flexion	Forward bending of the spinal bones. Example: Poses that bring the front of your torso toward your legs, such as Child's Pose
Extension	Backward bending of the spinal bones. Example: The movement required for backbends such as Cobra and Sphinx poses
Lateral side bending	The movement required to take you into side-bending yoga poses. Example: Crescent Moon Pose
Rotation	The movement for all yoga poses that involve a little or a lot of twisting of the spinal bones. Example: Easy Seated Twist

Movements of the Shoulder

MOVEMENT	DESCRIPTION
Flexion	Reaching the arm forward of the body and up overhead as far as it can go. As the upper arm bone moves in flexion, the shoulder blade slides around and up the side of the rib cage. Example: Bringing arms forward and up in Tree Pose
Extension	Reaching your arm back behind your body. As you do this, your shoulder blade slides down and back toward the spine. Example: Locust Pose. Also happens when you release arms from flexion. Example: Releasing arms from Tree Pose
Abduction	Taking arms from alongside your body out to your side (example: Warrior 2 Pose) or continuing through an out-to-the-side position all the way up to alongside your head (example: Arms Overhead Pose). Shoulder blade action is the same as in flexion.
Adduction	Taking your arm from overhead out to parallel with the floor or all the way down to your side (example: releasing your arms in Warrior 2 Pose) or crossing your arms in front of your body (example: your front arm in a seated twist).
External rotation	Rolling the upper arm bone out away from the midline of your body (the lower arm bones follow). Example: Turning your elbow creases and palms toward the ceiling in Relaxation Pose
Internal rotation	Rolling the upper arm bone in toward the midline of your body (the lower arm bones follow). Examples: Bringing the arms to Mountain Pose with Reverse Prayer position or elbows clasped behind your back

Movements of the Wrists

MOVEMENT	DESCRIPTION
Flexion	From arms straight out in front of you with palms down, bending wrist so the palm of your hand faces your chest. Rarely used in yoga poses, except in Arms Overhead with fingers interlaced and palms facing down.
Extension	From arms straight out in front of you with palms down, bending the wrists so the palms face away from you. Examples: Slight extension of wrists in Downward-Facing Dog Pose and 90-degree flexion in Dynamic Cat-Cow Pose

Abduction	From arms at sides with palms facing forward, moving the pinky sides of the hand away from your body.
Adduction	From arms at sides and palms facing forward, moving the pinky sides of hands toward the midline of your body.

Note on rotation: Although it feels like the wrist joints can rotate, this action actually comes from the forearm bones rolling over one another, not from any rotation of the wrist joint itself.

Movements of the Knees

MOVEMENT	DESCRIPTION
Flexion	Bending your knee (moving lower leg bones up and back toward upper leg). Examples: Moving front leg in standing poses into bent-knee position or bending both knees deeply, as in Hero Pose or Child's Pose
Extension	Starting from a bent knee position, straightening your knee (moving lower leg bones forward and away from upper leg). Examples: Straightening knee to exit Warrior 2 Pose, lifting back leg in Hunting Dog Pose, or moving into Downward-Facing Dog Pose from all fours
External rotation	When your knee is bent, rolling the lower leg bones outward, away from the midline (it rolls a small amount at the knee joint *only* when the knee is in flexion). Example: Movement of knee/lower leg bones in Cobbler's Pose, both seated and reclined
Internal rotation	When your knee is bent, rolling the lower leg bones in, toward the midline of your body (it can internally rotate a small amount *only* when the knee is in flexion). Example: Movement of knee/lower leg bones in Hero Pose

Movements of the Elbows

MOVEMENT	DESCRIPTION
Flexion	Bending your elbow (moving forearm toward upper arm). Example: From straight arms, bending upper arms into Prayer position
Extension	Straightening the elbow (moving forearm away from upper arm). Example: From Prayer position, releasing the arms into a straight position
Supination	Turning the forearms outward. You can do this movement with straight arms or elbows bent at any angle. Example: From arms at your sides in Mountain Pose, turning your forearms so palms face forward

Pronation   Turning the forearms inward. You can do this movement with straight arms or elbows bent at any angle. Example: From arms at your sides in Mountain Pose with palms facing your body, turning your forearms so your palms face behind you

Inverted Poses

In yoga, "inverting" means going upside down, even if you're just partly upside down. Any pose where your heart is higher than your head is considered an "inversion." There are three types of inverted poses:

1. Full inversion—Your heart is higher than your head, and your pelvis, legs, and feet are higher than your heart. The full inversions include Headstand, (Sirsasana), Shoulderstand (Salamba Sarvangasana), and Plow Pose (Halasana), as well as several challenging arm balances, such as Handstand (Adho Mukha Yrksasana)—none of which we're including in this book.

2. Partial inversion—Your heart and pelvis are above your head, but your feet are below your heart. This category includes Standing Forward Bend, Downward-Facing Dog Pose, and Widespread Standing Forward Bend (Prasarita Padottanasana). Standing Forward Bend and Downward-Facing Dog Pose are included in this book.

3. Gentle inversion—More gradual poses than the straight up and down inversions of heart directly over the head in partial and full inversions. In these poses, although your heart is higher than your head, it is only slightly higher. These poses include Legs Up the Wall Pose and Bridge Pose, both of which are included in this book. Because these two poses are very gentle, if you have hypertension or other conditions for which inverted poses are typically not recommended, you can give these poses a try, starting out with very short holds and gradually working up to longer holds over time.

NOTES

Chapter 1: What Is Yoga for Healthy Aging?

1. Nina Rook, "Comfort with Uncertainty," *Yoga for Healthy Aging* (blog), November 1, 2016, http://yogaforhealthyaging.blogspot.com/2016/11/comfort-with-uncertainty.html.
2. Juan Mascaró, trans., *The Bhagavad Gita* (London: Penguin, 2003), 13.
3. Stephen Mitchell, trans., *Bhagavad Gita: A New Translation* (New York: Harmony, 2002), 55.
4. B. K. S. Iyengar, *Yoga: The Path to Holistic Health* (New York: DK Publishing, 2013), 161.

Chapter 3: Yoga for Strength

1. Baxter Bell, "Stronger Now Than at 65: An Interview with Ellen Pechman," *Yoga for Healthy Aging* (blog), February 2, 2016, http://yogaforhealthyaging.blogspot.com/2016/02/stronger-now-than-at-65-interview-with.html.
2. Ibid.

Chapter 5: Yoga for Balance

1. Nina Zolotow, "Starting to Move Again, Part 2," *Yoga for Healthy Aging* (blog), April 17, 2014, http://yogaforhealthyaging.blogspot.com/2014/04/starting-to-move-again-part-2-progress.html.

Chapter 6: Yoga for Agility

1. Nina Rook, "Yoga-Given Agility," *Yoga for Healthy Aging* (blog), September 7, 2016, http://yogaforhealthyaging.blogspot.com/2016/09/yoga-given-agility.html.

Chapter 7: Heart and Cardiovascular System Health

1. Victor Dubin, "Low-Pressure Tactics: Using Yoga to Lower Blood Pressure," *Yoga for Healthy Aging* (blog), October 11, 2016, http://yogaforhealthyaging.blogspot.com/2016/10/low-pressure-tactics-using-yoga-to.html.
2. Ibid.
3. Ibid.

Chapter 8: Brain and Nervous System Health

1. Ram Rao, "Mental Exercise, Yoga and the Perfect Brain," *Yoga for Healthy Aging* (blog), April 16, 2014, http://yogaforhealthyaging.blogspot.com/2014/04/mental-exercise-yoga-and-perfect-brain.html.

Chapter 9: Stress Management

1. L/Cpl USMC, "Yoga and PTSD," *Yoga for Healthy Aging* (blog), October 12, 2016, http://yogaforhealthyaging.blogspot.com/2016/10/yoga-and-ptsd.html.
2. Nina Zolotow, "Keeping Your Cool: Stress Management and Equanimity," *Yoga for Healthy Aging* (blog), November 15, 2015, http://yogaforhealthyaging.blogspot.com/2015/11/keeping-your-cool-stress-management-and.html.
3. Rook, "Comfort with Uncertainty."
4. Kelly McGonigal, *The Willpower Instinct* (New York: Penguin, 2013), 24.

Chapter 10: Cultivating Equanimity

1. Mary Ann Avallone-O'Gorman, "After Hurricane Katrina," *Yoga for Healthy Aging* (blog), January 21, 2016, http://yogaforhealthyaging.blogspot.com/2016/01/after-hurricane-katrina.html.
2. Juan Mascaró, trans., *The Bhagavad Gita* (London: Penguin, 2003), 68.
3. B. K. S. Iyengar, trans., *Light on the Yoga Sūtras of Patañjali* (San Francisco: Thorsons, 1996), 147.
4. Rook, "Comfort with Uncertainty."

5. Edwin F. Bryant, trans., *The Yoga Sūtras of Patañjali: A New Edition, Translation, and Commentary* (New York: North Point Press, 2009), 10.

6. Ibid., 128.

7. Ram Rao, "Achieving Stillness in Turbulent Situations," *Yoga for Healthy Aging* (blog), January 29, 2013, http://yogaforhealthyaging .blogspot.com/2013/01/achieving-stillness-in-turbulent.html.

8. Baxter Bell, "The Power of Pranayama: Debbie's Story," *Yoga for Healthy Aging* (blog), November 3, 2016, http://yogaforhealthyaging .blogspot.com/2016/11/the-power-of-pranayama-debbies-story.html.

9. Jill Satterfield, "Recovering from Heart Surgery," *Yoga for Healthy Aging* (blog), September 8, 2016, http://yogaforhealthyaging.blogspot .com/2016/09/recovering-from-heart-surgery-interview.html.

Chapter 11: Yoga Philosophy

1. Henry David Thoreau, *Familiar Letters of Henry David Thoreau* (Charleston, SC: Nabu Press, 2012), 210.

2. Evelyn Zak, "Yoga for Recovery: Evelyn's Story," *Yoga for Healthy Aging* (blog), November 16, 2016, http://yogaforhealthyaging.blog-spot.com/2016/11/yoga-for-recovery-evelyns-story.html.

3. Ibid.

4. Mitchell, trans., *Bhagavad Gita*, 95.

5. Bryant, *The Yoga Sūtras of Patañjali*, 50.

6. Stephen Cope, *The Wisdom of Yoga* (New York: Bantam Books, 2006), 115.

7. Bryant, *The Yoga Sūtras of Patañjali*, 55.

8. Mitchell, trans., *Bhagavad Gita*, 55.

9. Bryant, *The Yoga Sūtras of Patañjali*, 255.

10. Mascaró, trans., *The Bhagavad Gita*, 13.

11. M. K. Gandhi, *The Bhagavad Gita According to Gandhi* (Blacksburg, VA: Wilder Publications, 2012), 10.

12. Mascaró, trans., *The Bhagavad Gita*, 18.

13. Mohandas K. Gandhi, *An Autobiography: The Story of My Experiments with Truth* (Boston: Beacon Press, 1957), 265.

14. Iyengar, trans., *Light on the Yoga Sūtras of Patañjali*, 46.

15. Georg Feuerstein, *Yoga: The Technology of Ecstasy* (New York: Jeremy P. Tarcher, 1989), 13.

16. Rook, "Comfort with Uncertainty."

17. Jill Satterfield, "Spiritual Sanity," *Yoga for Healthy Aging* (blog), August 14, 2014, http://yogaforhealthyaging.blogspot.com/2014/08/spiritual-sanity.html.

18. Iyengar, trans., *Light on the Yoga Sūtras of Patañjali*, 105 and 112.

19. Bryant, *The Yoga Sūtras of Patañjali*, 22.

20. T. K. V. Desikachar, trans., *The Heart of Yoga* (Rochester, VT: Inner Traditions, 199), 149.

21. Satterfield, "Spiritual Sanity."

22. Georg Feuerstein, trans., *The Deeper Dimensions of Yoga* (Boston, MA: Shambhala, 2003), 22.

23. B. K. S. Iyengar, *Light on Life: The Yoga Journey to Wholeness, Inner Peace, and Ultimate Freedom* (London: Rodale Books, 2008), 256.

24. Beth Gibbs, "Enough," *Yoga for Healthy Aging* (blog), December 2, 2015, http://yogaforhealthyaging.blogspot.com/2015/12/enough.html.

25. I. K. Taimni, *The Science of Yoga* (Wheaton, IL: Quest Books, 1961), 224.

26. T. K. V. Desikachar, *Health, Healing, and Beyond* (New York: North Point Press, 1998), 66.

27. Swami Jnaneshvara Bharati, "Yoga Sutras of Patanjali Interpretive Translation," PDF, www.swamij.com/pdf/yogasutrasinterpretive.pdf.

28. Gibbs, "Enough."

29. Mascaró, trans., *The Bhagavad Gita*, 64.

30. Feuerstein, trans., *The Yoga Tradition*, xxx.

INDEX OF POSES AND SEQUENCES

INDEX

abdominal conditions, 212, 222, 232,
    240, 246, 272, 291, 292
acid reflux disease, 238, 256, 291
active poses
    in balancing practice session, 140
    in Brain Health Practice, 124–125
    for cardiovascular health, 102
    holding, 16–17, 103
    overstretching in, 58
    props in, 19
    resting between, 22
    for strength, 34
activity, physical, 31, 47, 65–66
acute stress, 132–133, 137
addiction, 188
afflictions, five, 195–196
agility, 7, 11, 81–82
    aging and, 84
    balance and, 70, 90
    skills needed for, 82–83
    yogic techniques for, 86–88
aging
    agility and, 84
    balance and, 68–70
    brain and, 113–114
    cardiovascular system and, 97–98
    compressed morbidity and, 6–7
    definition of, 4
    equanimity and, 8
    flexibility and, 51–53
    independence and, 7, 8

    learning and, 119
    Nancy's story, 3–4, 6, 7, 8, 199
    nervous system and, 115
    seven pillars of, 5, 128
    and strength, role in, 30–33
ahimsa. See nonviolence (*ahimsa*)
alternate nostril breathing (*nadi
    sodhana*), 78, 181–182
Alzheimer's disease, 109, 111–112,
    114
anemia, 97
anxiety
    blood lactate and, 136
    chronic stress and, 117, 132,
        133–134
    contraindications for, 291
    poses prescribed for, 218, 224, 230,
        260, 262, 278
arthritis
    facet joint, 292
    flexibility and, 48, 53
    leg strength and, 34
    muscle strength and, 30
    poses prescribed for, 216, 242, 252
    shoulder and arm, postures for, 210
asanas. See poses (*asanas*)
asthma, 172, 291
autonomic nervous system, 113,
    115, 128–130, 134. *See also*
        parasympathetic nervous system;
        sympathetic nervous system

ABOUT THE CONTRIBUTORS

Baxter Bell, MD, C-IAYT, eRYT500

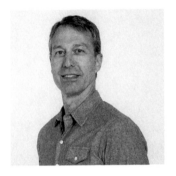

Cofounder of the *Yoga for Healthy Aging* blog, Baxter is a medical doctor and a medical acupuncturist as well as a certified yoga teacher and yoga therapist. Baxter practiced as a family physician from 1989 to 2000. Then, in 2001, he completed the 18-month, 680-hour Advanced Studies Program at Piedmont Yoga Studio in Oakland, California, with Richard Rosen, Rodney Yee, Mary Paffard, and Patricia Sullivan. In 2000, he completed his 300-hour medical acupuncture training. In 2017, he was certified as a yoga therapist by the International Association of Yoga Therapists.

Based in Oakland, California, Baxter was director of the Deep Yoga Teacher Training at Piedmont Yoga Studio for seven years and is currently serving as an adjunct faculty member on teacher training programs and therapeutic yoga trainings around the country. He teaches locally in the San Francisco Bay Area, offering regular yoga classes to the general public as well as specialty classes for those with back pain and adults with disabilities, and teaches workshops and retreats worldwide with an emphasis on yoga for healthy aging and how yoga can be used therapeutically to improve health and well-being. He also combines his experience as a family physician with his training in medical acupuncture in his complementary medical practice in Oakland, where he focuses on acupuncture and therapeutic yoga. He is featured in the *Yoga Journal: Yoga for Stress* DVD as well as on the Practice Channel at YogaUOnline.com. To find out more about Baxter or to contact him, visit BaxterBell.com, and to view his instructional videos (including for many of the poses in this book), visit his YouTube channel "Baxter Bell Yoga."

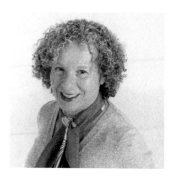

Nina Zolotow, RYT500

Editor in Chief of the *Yoga for Healthy Aging* blog, Nina is a yoga writer as well as a certified yoga teacher and a longtime yoga practitioner. Based in Berkeley, California, Nina's areas of expertise are yoga for healthy aging, yoga for emotional well-being (including yoga for stress, insomnia, depression, and anxiety), and cultivating equanimity. She completed the three-year teacher training program at The Yoga Room in Berkeley, has studied yoga therapy with Shari Ser and Bonnie Maeda, and is especially influenced by the teachings of Donald Moyer. She has also studied extensively with Rodney Yee, and she is inspired by the teachings of Patricia Walden on yoga for emotional healing. She teaches workshops and series classes on yoga for healthy aging, yoga for emotional well-being, yoga for stress, yoga for better sleep, home practice, and cultivating equanimity. Nina is the coauthor, with Rodney Yee, of two books on yoga: *Moving Toward Balance* and *Yoga: The Poetry of the Body*, and she's the author of numerous articles on yoga and alternative medicine.

To stay in touch with both Baxter and Nina, visit the *Yoga for Healthy Aging* blog at YogaforHealthyAging.blogspot.com, where you can read their recent posts, search the archives, or subscribe to their e-mail service that delivers articles to you five days a week. You can also follow them on Facebook by liking their *Yoga for Healthy Aging* page.

About the Photographer

Melina Meza, 500-ERYT, BS Nutrition. Melina is an Oakland, California-based photographer, yoga teacher, and ayurvedic health educator. She received her yoga training from Dr. Robert Svoboda, Gary Kraftsow, Scott Blossom, Sarah Powers, Tias Little, and Jin Sung, and is a certified Yoga for Healthy Aging teacher. Her BS in nutrition is from Bastyr University, and she received Ayurvedic Health Educator certification from the California College of Ayurveda. From 1997 to 2011, she taught yoga full time at 8 Limbs Yoga Centers in Seattle, Washington, and she is currently the codirector of their 200- and 500-hour Teacher Training programs. Melina has been exploring the art and science of yoga and nutrition for over twenty years, and she developed Seasonal Vinyasa, an innovative, multidisciplinary approach to well-being. She is also the author of three *Art of Sequencing* yoga books. To find out more or to contact Melina, visit MelinaMeza.com.

About the Model

Sandy Carmellini, CIYT-1000, ERYT-500. Sandy is both a certified Iyengar Yoga teacher and a certified Yoga for Healthy Aging teacher, and she has been teaching yoga in the San Francisco Bay Area since 1998. She was a devoted student for many years of Donald Moyer, who is now retired. She continues to study regularly with Sri H. S. Arun from Bangalore, and she travels to India regularly to deepen her studies with him and with the Iyengar family. She opened her studio, Brentwood Yoga Center, in Brentwood, California, in 2008. To find out more or to contact Sandy, visit BrentwoodYogaCenter.com.